Book Reviews

Buildings are becoming unhealthier every day. Poor and contaminated building materials are all around. Sick Buildings are actually one of the root causes of our diseases. I think such a book will help Architects, Builders and Vastu Advisers in understanding the clear relationship between building-design and health.

–Padmashree Dr. J.R. Bhalla
Former President–Council of Architects

I have seen the contents of the book on Sick Building Syndrome that Prof. Dr. Puri and Dr. Mehra are writing. I would like to admire and encourage such a title because most of the diseases that relate to a building are not diagnosed at the root-level and hence, the root cause of the disease remains unknown. Such awareness will help people at large to live a healthy life style.

–Padmashree Dr. S.K. Sama
Former Chairman–Sir Ganga Ram Hospital

In order to live a healthy life, awareness about Sick Building Syndrome would help people a lot. In western countries, this is a popular subject and most of the people are aware of Sick Building Syndrome. I hope *SBS* becomes popular in India as well.

–Dr. P.S. Rana
Ex-Chairman, HUDCO, New Delhi

I liked the contents of the book Dr. Puri and Dr. Mehra are writing; a great subject. I think this book can help everyone at large in improving their living conditions.

–Dr. Nalini Kaul
Director, Medanta

Do You Know?

Your Building Can Make You Sick!!!

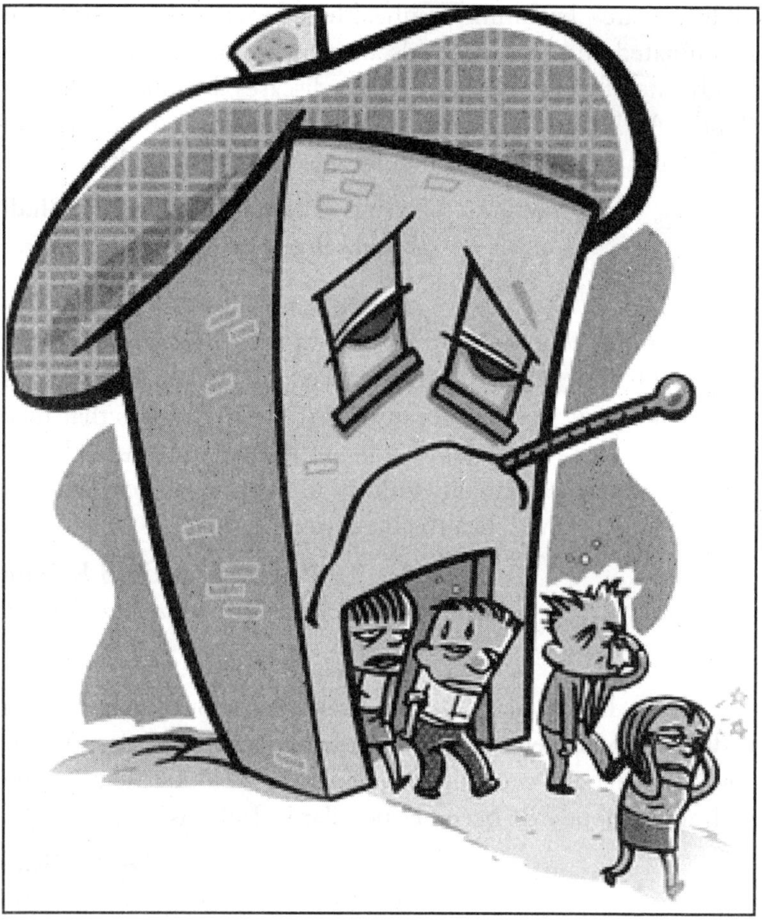

Make Your Building Healthy and Nature Friendly

Sick Building Syndrome

A Complete Guide To Sick Building Issues—Solutions From Vastu Science

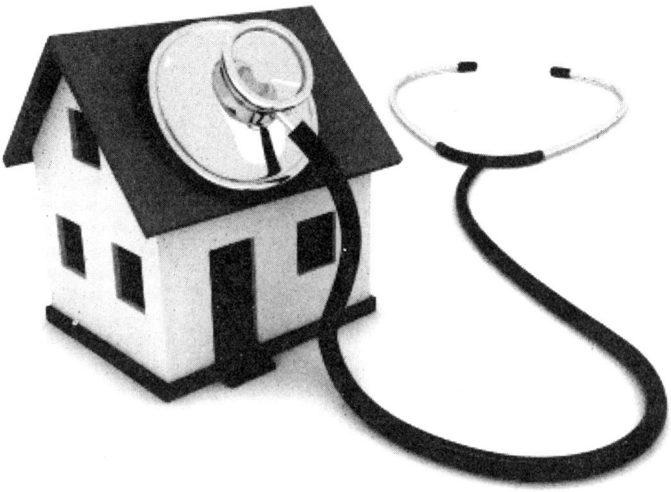

Prof. Dr. B.B. Puri

Dr. R.M. Mehra

BOOKS FOR ALL

Delhi

First Published 2015

ISBN 13: 978-81-7386-311-0
ISBN 10: 81-7386-311-3

Published by
BOOKS FOR ALL
A-6, Second Floor, Nimri Commercial Centre,
Ashok Vihar Phase-4, Delhi - 110 052 (India)
Tel.: +91 11 2730 2453 Fax: 011 4706 1936
website: www.LPPindia.com
e-mail: info@LPPindia.com

Printed at
D.K. Fine Art Press Pvt. Ltd.
Delhi

PRINTED IN INDIA

Contents

1
Introduction

What is Sick Building Syndrome

A human body is a living organism or structure, embodied with energies in and around, with self maintained systems (physiology) running by themselves to maintain the organism. Similarly a building is also an enclosed vibrating structure with embodied energies in and around with partially self created systems & process primarily supported by forces of nature. Every structure is an enclosed space or embodied spatial form surcharged with energies within.

A building is like a human body in many aspects. Human body can become sick if it is exposed to unhealthy environment. Over exposure to carbon monoxide, sulphur dioxide, negative radiations, energies, or unhealthy air with organic and inorganic contaminations can drive a living organism towards sickness. Similarly a building which is exposed to similar unhealthy conditions can become sick and make the occupants sick. If a building becomes sick for long durations, the internal bioclimate of the building which is self created self maintained systems gets badly affected. As a result the whole internal system (internal bioclimate) of the building becomes unhealthy. When the complete anatomy and physiology (structure and its functioning) of the building gets affected, it is termed as SICK BUILDING.

If 20% or more of the building's occupants complain of such problems as headache, eye irritation, nausea, sore throats, dry or itchy skin, sinus congestion, nose irritation, fatigue and dizziness etc. for more than two weeks, it may indicate Sick Building Syndrome. It is also described as human health conditions where infections linger, caused by exposure to toxins and contaminants within a building as a result of poor ventilation, lack of natural sunlight, negative radiations, energies, stresses and aggressions. It is an Ill-health or discomfort caused by a structure's design and/or the materials used to construct it.

The **United States Environmental Protection Agency** (**USEPA**) describes the term "Sick Building Syndrome (SBS) as situations in which building occupants experience acute health and comfort effects that appear to be linked to time spent in a building, but no specific illness or cause can be identified. The complaints may be localized in a particular room or zone, or may be widespread throughout the building. In contrast, the term "building related illness" (BRI) is used when symptoms of diagnosable illness are identified and can be attributed directly to airborne building contaminants."

The Environmental Illness Resource describes Sick Building Syndrome as a broad label that covers a range of symptoms thought to be triggered when the sufferer spends time in a particular building. Symptoms range from specific symptoms such as itchy eyes, skin rashes, and nasal allergy symptoms, to more vague symptoms such as fatigue, aches and pains, and sensitivity to odours.

The term "Sick Building Syndrome", was first coined in the 1970s, and its recognition at this time may in part be attributable to the increasing presence of electronic equipment and other factors. It is used when the symptoms of a significant number of people occupying a particular building, are associated with their presence in that building. In most cases Sick Building Syndrome occurs in office buildings, although it may also occur in other communal buildings such as schools and apartment buildings.

Wikipedia describes Sick Building Syndrome (SBS) is a combination of ailments (a syndrome) associated with an individual's place of work (office building) or residence.

Wiktionary has described Sick Building Syndrome as adverse environmental conditions in a building that pose a health risk to its occupants; the symptoms experienced by people who work there.

In our opinion Sick Building Syndrome is a complex problem created by multiple factors both physical and non physical in nature, affecting not just the physical but also the mental, emotional, intellectual and spiritual comfort and balance of the occupants. It is not just created through poor indoor air quality and poor building materials as mostly known but is also affected by many other factors combininly creating unhealthy internal bioclimate including holistic factors too.

As seen above that most of the agencies have related sickness of building mostly with indoor air. But there are some others as well who have also related it with electromagnetic pollution, negative radiations and other adverse conditions of the building. It is important to note that Sick Building Syndrome is a situation created by multiple factors making it sick or healthy. The factors can be classified as internal factors and external factors. Both external and internal environment have a strong impact on the mental and physical health of the occupants. All the external factors including air quality, humidity, dust, sound levels, natural light levels and location etc have a strong impact on the physiology or functioning of automatic systems of the building. Similarly the internal factors are also equally affective like geopathic stress, indoor air quality, internal light levels, negative radiations, out gassing from building materials, electromagnetic fields and so on.

Vastu Science, ancient Indian science of architecture talks about building construction, building materials, environmental quality and higher standard of living through energy efficient and sustainable habitats. People have lived longer and healthier lives in structures which were merely nature supportive. Our ancient architects knew the art and science of wise creation of buildings. Such structures are still evidently visible to learn from our glorious past. The term like Sick Building Syndrome is today's problem. It is a problem created through unwise planning, poor ideology, structures, materials and primarily lack of knowledge about sensitive aspects of life and building.

There have been some scholars in ancient and modern architecture who have even added that Sick Building Syndrome is some total of both scientific and holistic constraints of building or poor hygienic living conditions. A building may have holistic defects if it has not been designed as per the laws of nature. Therefore Sick Building Syndrome is a much wider term than it seems. It is much detailed because it is not just unhealthy conditions created by unhealthy air but combination of external and internal scientific and holistic factors.

Health and home has a close relationship. People get affected by the environment they live in. For instance if a couple stays in a very congested lane of a congested market in a metropolitan with very high pollution levels, little natural light, high noise levels and internal environment consisting of high electromagnetic field, contaminating materials and geopathic stress. If such a couple moves to a hill station where the building is located on a healthy location with green trees all around. In such a case the couple will find a drastic difference in their life and lifestyle. They would find a better improved mental and physical health. Such is the affect of environment on the occupants.

Causes of Sick Building Syndrome

Although in many cases the exact mechanism by which a building, or substances within the building are causing the occupants to become ill is unknown, the problem areas can usually be identified and remedial action can be taken. In many Sick Building Syndrome cases poor building design, maintenance, and operation of the structure's ventilation system may be at fault. The cross ventilation system in particular is often found to be at the heart of the problem, and can itself be a source of irritants. In addition, a poor ventilation system can result in a build-up of pollutants within the building, in which case the indoor environment can often have air quality much lower than the outdoor air. Factors such as architecture or interior design may also interfere with efficient functioning of ventilation systems. Essentially poor design and maintenance of the ventilation system can enhance the negative health effects.

It has been suggested that very low levels of specific pollutants, such as VOCs, that are present inside a building may act to cause symptoms of illness. The chemical industry is not strictly regulated and majority of chemicals have not been tested for health effects. Today the scientists are active in finding even minute negative effects of a chemical emission as such collective gross emissions from multiple chemicals may be highly dangerous. Example of such a massacre is Union carbon factory Bhopal.

The symptoms of SBS are likely the result of a combination of factors. Many of the symptoms can be related either to the known toxic effects of high levels of certain chemicals emitted from a recognizable source within or outside the building. Some of the prominent causes of Sick Building Syndrome are mentioned below:

- ✓ Poor Indoor Air Quality & Ventilation
- ✓ Lack of Sunlight & Seasonal affective Disorder
- ✓ Electromagnetic Pollution
- ✓ Noise Pollution
- ✓ Unhealthy Building Material & Multiple Chemical Sensitivity
- ✓ Construction Bye passing Vastu Principles
- ✓ Extreme Climatic Conditions & Sick Building Syndrome
- ✓ Geopathic Stress & Land Degradation
- ✓ Poor Surroundings & Vegetation
- ✓ Furniture & Unhealthy Internal environment

Symptoms of Sick Building Syndrome

The symptoms of Sick Building may vary conditionally. The symptoms depend on the type of emission and the people affected by such emissions. In general conditions there can be a long list of problems that people may face during their stay in the building. Several sick occupants may complain individual symptoms which may not appear to be connected. Generally the symptoms may not appear as soon as the occupant leaves the building. Although there may be a mild lingering affect throughout. In fact in sensitive individuals there can be long-term health effects too.

Buildings often contain a lot of hidden and unapproachable spaces within the building. Such spaces may include attic, crawlspace, and drop-ceiling spaces etc. Such spaces suffer from absence of infiltration and inadequate ventilation. It is technically referred to as "Stagnation". The symptoms of Sick Building Syndrome are mentioned below:

Sick Building Syndrome Symptoms	
• Burning and watering eyes and nose • Burning in trachea • Cancer • Chronic fatigue • CNS (Central Nervous System) tremors or loss of balance • Debilitating fibromyalgia (muscle cramps and joint pain) • Depression • Dizziness • Dry, itchy skin • Exhaustion after normal activity • Hair loss • Headaches • Heart Palpitations • Hoarseness, cough, sore throat • Inability to concentrate	• Irritability • Itchy granulomous pimples • Miscarriages • Nausea • Neuropathy (loss of sensation in extremities) • Nosebleeds • Pregnancy Problems • Sensitivity to odors • Serious edema (swelling of legs, trunk, ankles) • Shortness of breath upon mild exertion (e.g. walking) • Tremors • Weight gain • Wellness When Away From Building

Unhealthy Environment & Diseases

Mind and Body

A question comes to the mind more and often. What is the relationship between the mind and the body? Philosophers and scientists have been debating on this topic. Mind is an abstract term used for the workings of the brain. Brain is one the most important parts of the body. It is directly connected by nerves to all other parts of the body. Whatever is going on "mentally" inside a person is also going on physically, and vice versa. It is a fact that most of the time we are not conscious of the activities going on in our brain. We are conscious only of the effects of that activity. This is why it is considered that although it is part of the body still it is apart from the body.

Why Mental and Physical Diseases

According to "Flanders Dunbar" it is more important to know what kind of person has the disease rather than to know what kind of disease the person has. It is more important to understand the psyche of a person so as to know the root cause of the disease. For example if a person is fatigued, it will reduce his ability to withstand any stress and if the person is stressed it will reduce his ability to withstand any physical disease. These are therefore known as psychosomatic disorders.

Generally diseases are born out of unhealthy living or living conditions. Now it is up to us to understand and clearly define healthy and unhealthy living. If we intend to live a healthy life, we must understand clearly how to stay healthy and create healthy building environment. In lot of cases it has been clearly concluded that Building and its environment was the ROOT CAUSE of the problem. A person is most affected by the environment. The overall environment is a result of temperature, light, sound, indoor air quality, construction material, furniture, electronic gadgets, orientation and direction etc.

Just to emphasize on the relationship between an unhealthy environment and diseases, some of the examples are stated below:

- *Unhealthy interior material* can cause multiple chemical sensitivity.
- *Imbalance* in the air can cause depression, irritability and rashes etc
- *Radon* gas emissions can even cause cancer
- Over exposure to *sound* can cause palpitation, blood vessel constriction, and adrenaline rush and pupil dilation.
- *Unhealthy furniture* can cause repetitive strain injury, backache, pain in shoulders and neck, mid back and lower back pain and even stress and tension.
- *Contaminations* in the air can cause chronic bronchitis, sneezing, watery eyes, coughing, dizziness, lethargy, fever, humidifier fever and digestive problems.
- Exposure to too much of *light* can cause skin related diseases
- *Unhealthy plants* can cause allergies and infections
- *Geopathic Stress* can cause lowering down of immunization system, cramps and inflammations.
- *Electro magnetic pollution* can cause insomnia and migraine.
- *Fungus* (wuchereria bancrofti) can cause elephantiasis (swelling of foot)
- *Bacteria* can cause encephalitis and syphilis
- Lack of *Cosmo telluric channel* can cause uneasiness and lack of freshness

The impact of overall environment on the human body is explained through the below mentioned diagram.

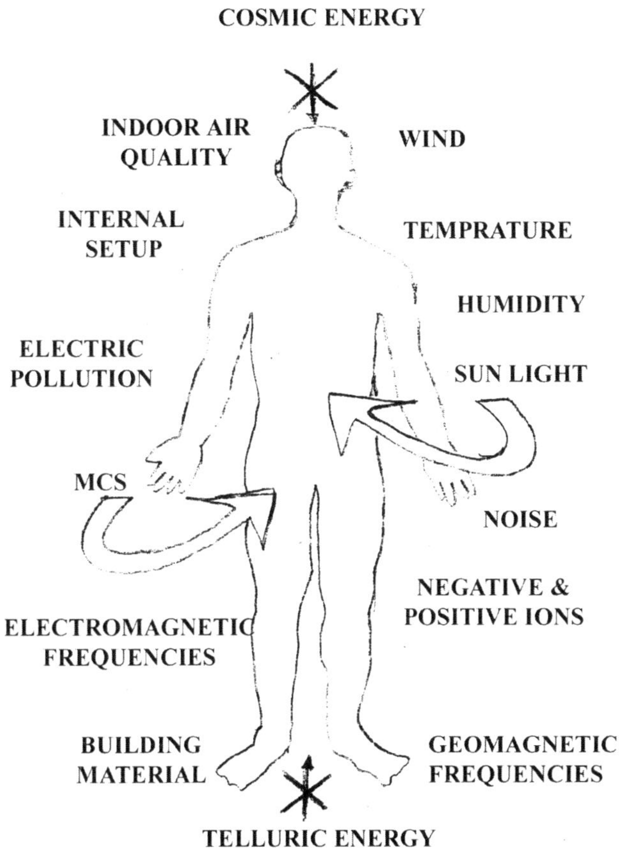

Impact of overall Environment on Human body

The mental and physical health of the occupants depends a lot on the environment. Healthy environment can help a person grow better both mentally and physically. Various diseases can also occur due to unhealthy conditions. A small description of the problems that can happen due to environmental conditions is given below:

Major Depressive Episode

A person may get into psychological trauma and later into a major depressive episode due to unhealthy environment. The person who is entering into a depressive episode undergoes profound changes in most aspects of his or her functioning. It is not just mood but also motivation, thinking, physical and motor functioning that gets affected. The following are the characteristic features of the major depressive episode:

1. *Depressed mood*

Generally people living in depressive environment report sadness or unhappiness, ranging from a mild sadness to total hopelessness. Moderately depressed people go for frequent crying spells; they feel like crying but cannot. Deeply depressed people consider their condition as irreversible; they cannot help themselves, nor can anyone possibly help them. This way of thinking has been characterized as the helplessness-hopelessness syndrome.

2. *Loss of Pleasure*

Loss of Pleasure means lack of interest in usual activities. The absence of pleasure is known as anhedonia. The person does not find interest in doing anything for example going to temple, eating food or playing guitar etc. The patients experience a complete "paralysis of will" -an inability even to get out of bed in the morning.

3. *Disturbance of appetite*

People who suffer from unhealthy and depressive environment may face a loss of appetite followed by a loss in weight. As stated earlier such people lose interest in food and it does not taste good to them anymore. There is a lot of disturbance in diet patterns too.

4. *Sleep disturbances*

Insomnia is an extremely common feature of depression. It generally happens in case of posttraumatic stress disorder. The most common characteristic is that people awake too early in the morning and then feel being unable to get back to sleep. It has also been noticed that such people suffer from trouble in falling asleep initially, they may awaken repeatedly throughout the night or they have a disturbed sleep throughout.

5. *Psychomotor retardation or agitation*

In case of agitation, the patient suffers from a massive fatigue and shows little spontaneous activity. The posture is generally stooped, movement is slow and deliberate and the speech is low and halting with long pauses before answering.

6. *Loss of energy*

Patients suffering from stress, depression and unhealthy environment are found to have low energy levels. The occupant's motivation level goes down and it is accompanied by a sharply reduced energy level. Even without working the occupant feels exhausted all the time.

7. *Feeling of Worthlessness and Guilt*

Unhealthy Building environment can make the occupants feel worthless and full of guilt. They find maximum negatives within themselves like lack of intelligence, physical attractiveness, health, and social skills. They find themselves loosing love, material goods, money, or may be prestige. They portray a kind of insecurity and personal inadequacy.

8. Difficulties in thinking

In depression, mental processes are usually found to be slowed down. The occupants tend to be indecisive and they often report difficulties in thinking, concentrating, and remembering. This is a common problem found with all age groups but old age is prominently noticeable in a depressive environment.

Environmental relaxation affects the psychological conditions of an individual.

Therefore in order to create a healthy body with a healthy mind one must concentrate on creating a healthy environment.

2

Vastu Science

Science of Ancient Architecture (Vedic Architecture)

Lets learn from our glorious past

VASTU is a science of harmonious manifestation of energy into matter or vice versa. It is a technical study of harmonious balancing of human energies with natural energies. It is set of laws oriented to align maximum benefits from a micro climatic condition and a building structure.

Vastu Science is a study of life within a defined space or the study of relationship between the occupants and building in context to land, Location and environment. All the five factors should always be in harmony.

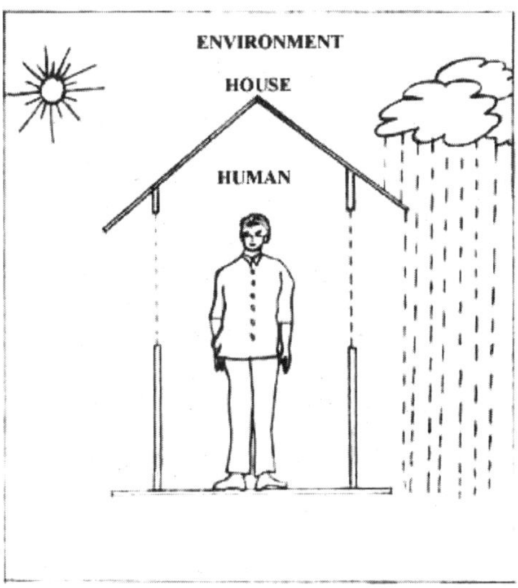

HEALTHY ENVIRONMENT MEANS A PERFECT INTEGRATION OF HUMAN HOUSE AND ENVIRONMENT

Vastu means Harmony with Nature

Occupant-To understand life of occupants in a building, it is essential to understand their psychology, behavioral patterns and generic disease pattern. The mind, body relationship needs to be clearly understood.

Building-To understand building from Vastu perspective, one must look at structure, architecture and interiors from directional perspective.

Land-Vastu emphasizes a lot on land selection. The land should have high bearing capacity and should also be fertile.

Location-The impact of location is given prime importance in Vastu.

Environment-The impact of both internal and external environment is strongly taken into consideration while implying Vastu.

Vastu means aligning a building with the laws of nature. It is perfect harmony between nature and building with the help of its five elements. Our ancient architects knew the art and science of creating energy efficient sustainable buildings. Now days we hear of Green Building, but in India people have always been living in Green Buildings. It is because of a rat race to reduce cost, fancy looks and changed priorities that people are facing problems of sick buildings. There are four directions north, south, east, west and four corners north east, south east, south west and north west. There are two vertical directions as well. All the directions and corners have their own specific characteristics. The objective of Vastu Science is to construct buildings with spiritual connect, which further helps the occupants to connect with themselves.

Scientific Approach to Vastu

Laws of nature

Whenever we talk about VASTU, we refer to cardinal directions. But in actual sense VASTU is an energy based science. It is basically harmonization of energies in and around the building. VASTU has scientific fundamentals which are universal in nature and can be proved. VASTU emphasizes on staying in harmony with the laws of nature. The movement of Sun, Moon & Earth, effect of celestial bodies, cosmo telluric channel, geo energies, climate, wind & other natural phenomena's affect our life drastically. The energies and vibrations around us have subtle impact on the body.

Vastu & Sun

Sun being the centre of the solar system, governs multiple forces in it. It affects our life immensely. It is known that in summer sun rises from northeast east, in equinox from east and in winters from southeast east. Similarly it sets in northwest west in summer, west in equinox and southwest west in winters. That is why we see longer days than nights in summer.

The fixed time of sunrise is morning whereby the fixed place of sunrise is east. Similarly the fixed time of sunset is evening whereby the fixed place of sunset is west. At the noon time the Sun is always in South with highest heat and glare. The most interesting phenomena is to observe morning in context to east, noon in context to south and evening in context to west. The most sensitive issues of life and connect are lying in connect with nature.

When we observe sunrise we notice high level of thermal and visual comfort in northeast throughout the day. The sun moves from northeast and slowly reaches east which is the permanent place of sun rise throughout the year. It is also important to understand, what people feel, at the time of sunrise. People, who see sunrise frequently, feel active, energetic, positive and fresh throughout the day. It is also seen that people develop better concentration and connectivity levels at the time of sunrise. Now if a building has adequate opening in north east & east, the morning rays of the sun enter into the room through windows and doors and create a permanent positive environment inside. It is not just thermal comfort, visual comfort, value of light, cool air, less noise and cool albedo but infact a complete connect of self with nature. Sun also makes the northeast & east part of the building active, energetic, positive, full of concentration and connectivity. This means if the building is balanced as per the laws of nature due to adequate openings in east & north east of the building will be active, energetic & certainly positive.

Sun moves and reaches southeast; almost by noon (time varies). At this point of time sun creates an irritant and unbearable heat. But the positive part of the rays of the sun is that they are disinfectant. The sunlight has high level of heat & energy that makes it competent enough to be disinfectant.

Sun reaches southwest of the building in the early evening. West direction is the direction of setting sun which is stable, relaxing and restful. Sun does not reach North therefore they turn out to be cool zones with cool light. North direction enjoys indirect cool and diffused light of sun. It is a place for day time rooms as it is blessed with thermal and visual comfort throughout the day. Green Building Criteria's (GRIHA- Criteria 13&14) emphasize on thermal and visual comfort in context to directions.

It is observed that even on the grounds of sun various room placements in a building can be done. The most important observation is creation of internal environment by Nature, and replicated impact on occupants. The objective of VASTU science is to give best to each functionality or use in a particular area for example concentration in study room, connectivity in prayer room, natural & disinfectant environment in kitchen, comfort and relaxed environment in bed room and contamination free environment in bathroom & toilet. This would improve the performance level of each activity and generate better level of efficiency with good results.

Solar Energy & Vastu

Solar energy is the energy, heat and light from Sun. The Earth receives 174 petawatts (PW) of incoming solar radiation (isolation) at the upper atmosphere. Approximately 30% is reflected back to space while the rest is absorbed by clouds, oceans and land masses. The spectrum of solar light at the Earth's surface is mostly spread across the visible and near-infrared ranges with a small part in the near-ultraviolet.

The total solar energy absorbed by Earth's atmosphere, oceans and land masses is approximately 3,850,000 exajoules (EJ) per year. The amount of solar energy reaching the surface of the planet is so vast that in one year it is about twice as much as will ever be obtained from all of the Earth's non-renewable resources of coal, oil, natural gas, and mined uranium combined.

Solar energy can be harnessed in different levels around the world. Depending on a geographical location the closer to the equator the more "potential" solar energy is available. VASTU emphasizes on creating solar efficient buildings which conserve energy and are green as well.

Cosmic Energy & Vastu

In cosmology, cosmic energy is a form of electromagnetic radiation filling the universe. With a radio telescope, there is a faint background glow, almost exactly the same in all directions, that is not associated with any star, galaxy, or other object. This glow is strongest in the microwave region of the radio spectrum, hence the name cosmic microwave background radiation. The cosmic radiations fill the whole universe with the ambient energy it has. VASTU as a science removes obstacles in the path of cosmic energy and building and fills the building with maximum cosmic radiations. Environmental Aggression may occur due to absence of adequate cosmic channel.

Magnetic Energy & Earth

The Earth acts as a giant magnet with opposing poles at the north and south. There is a flow of magnetism from North Pole to south pole. Its geomagnetic field (GMF) changes constantly, mostly due to the effects of solar radiation. The sun emits cosmic rays, which form a solar wind, a torrent of radiation, which bombards the Earth. The solar wind is made up of positively and negatively charged particles, which separate when they hit the Earth's magnetic field. Vastu Science manifests the best use of magnetic flow to enhance better efficiency, comfort and energy within the occupants.

The Earth Grid and Earth Net

Two German medical practitioners, Hartmann and Curry, have characterized the earth's GMF as being bundled in strips which cover the earth. The Hartmann global earth grid consists of a series of 4 inches to 9 inch thick invisible radioactive walls running from north to south, intersected by other strips running from east to west. The lines may also be influenced by the amount of interference and turbulence by present in the local environment. The curry net has wider bands running northeast to southwest and northwest to southeast which consist of 'standing waves', extending out from the earth's centre.

The junction points are called 'NODES'. Both curry and Hartmann grids present on the land have strong impact on human anatomy & psychology. Ancient Architects were wise in selecting appropriate land. They could detect the deformities in the land. The furniture layout was specifically kept the grid in mind if it is there. It was ensured that the occupants were not positioned over the grids.

Geopathic Stress & Vastu

Geo means Earth and Pathos means suffering. Geopathic Stress means suffering from the negative vibrations of the earth which causes stress in the form of illness. Geopathic Stress is the Earth's vibrations which rise up through the Earth and are distorted by weak electromagnetic fields created by certain mineral concentrations, fault lines and underground cavities, subterranean running water, and many more. The vibration distorted becomes abnormally high and harmful to living organisms. Geopathic Stress is the term used for natural or man-made energies emanating from the earth and which are detrimental to human health. Geopathology refers to influences originating from the soil that cause illness.

Other than the influences of the sun and other planets, the earth's GMF can also be affected by ground water movement. Faults in the earth's crust can increase neutron radiation from the core of the earth. These neutrons may be slowed down by the presence of underground water and become low-energy, thermal neutrons which can cause cell degeneration in organisms. The friction produced by the flow of water in underground channels formed by sand and gravel beds can also induce electromagnetic fields. Zones that are capable of causing ill. Students can refer to the researches submitted to the university on Geopathic Stress.

Geomagnetic field disturbances have been linked to cardiovascular diseases, and to changes in the central nervous system. The morphology and functioning of internal organs and the physiological and biochemical processes of animals get affected. They can affect blood clotting times and exacerbate the effects of other illnesses. By exposing us to changes in the GMF, building over, or close to, geomagnetic anomalies like geological faulting can affect our health. This applies even when the anomalies are deep below the surface of the earth. The deterioration in health associated with living in such a zone has been termed 'Geopathogenic stress' (or 'geopathic stress'). Our ancient architects have again been wiser in selecting suitable land for the occupants.

In case of stressed land natural herbal remedies were used for the land. Such remedies are also stated in Vedic Books of Architecture.

Impact of Poor Location

VASTU has always given a lot of importance to location and their effect on a building and its environment. Below mentioned are poor locations for a residence:

- Factory – (Contamination)
- Garbage Bin – (Contamination)
- Crowded Markets – (Noise Pollution)
- Hospital – (Contamination)
- Cremation Ground – (Contamination)

Five Element Theory

VASTU is a science discovered by our great saints and sages to make human beings more happy and prosperous in their homes, shops, factories and buildings.

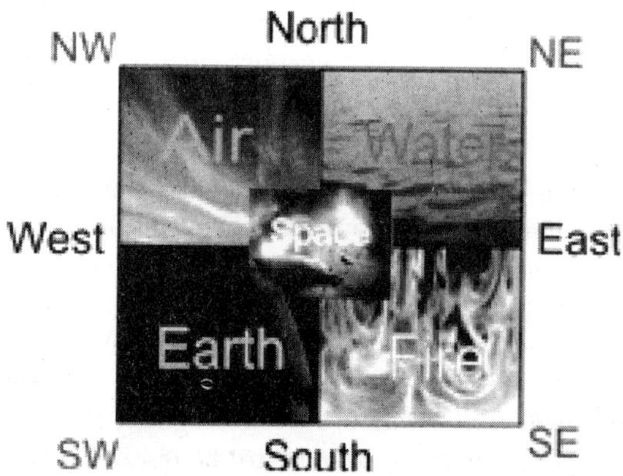

Earth, Water, Fire, Air and Sky are Five elements

Whole world including the human body comprises of five essential elements, i.e., earth, water, fire, air and sky. The principles of "VASTU" are mainly dependent on the arrangement and balancing of these five elements in their proper order and proportions so that the humans can have better living conditions in a place in which they live or work.

The principles of "VASTU" also keep in view the cosmic influence of the Sun, its light and heat, the direction of the wind, the magnetic influence of the earth and influence of cosmos and various other heavenly bodies on our planet earth. **As per Vastu Science balance of five elements is essential in a**

building and a body too. If there is a imbalance of five elements within or around the building, it can lead to ill health for the occupants.

- **WATER-NE**
- **FIRE-SE**
- **EARTH-SW**
- **AIR-NW**
- **SPACE-Centre**

FIRE

Fire, the Sun and Solar Energy

The sun's energy drives the photosynthesis of plants. The sun also enables our bodies to synthesis vitamin D by acting on the oils of our skin. Without vitamin D our body cannot assimilate calcium, phosphorus and other minerals, resulting in rickets, tooth decay, osteoporosis and retarded growth in children as well as muscular weakness and premature aging. The sun also contributes to some of the stellar cosmic radiation which arrives on earth. Most of the energy supplied to modern industry and our homes is derived from oil, petroleum, coal and natural gas, which are finite resources. Fire plays an important role in our lives. The fire element is placed in the southeast of the plot or building.

EARTH

Soil is a very precious resource, which is being wasted all over the world. It originates from the rock that makes up the earth's crust, a mixture of granite, sedimentary and metamorphic rock, over a period of 200 to 1200 years.

How soil and rock affect our health?

Soil and ground water, through natural processes, sometimes generate radio active pollutants, which can affect health. Uranium, occurring naturally in soil and rock, breaks down over millions of years to reach a stable state as lead. About halfway along uranium's decay chain, an element known as radon 222 forms.

Soil deficiencies

Many soils in the world are deficient in phosphorus, nitrogen and the trace elements copper and zinc. Most deficiencies are counteracted artificially with fertilizers but some experts suspect that something is lacking in the quality of vegetation produced on chemically fertilized soils.

Soil Abuse

The most serious problem of all is that of soil that has been rendered totally useless by the dumping of toxic chemicals or their leaching on to the ground water. Other forms of soil abuse arise from leaking storage tanks or pipelines and old stock-drenching sites.

Soil pH

The degree of acidity and alkalinity in soils (as well as their mineral element content) has a marked effect on plant growth, and hence on the availability of those nutrients upon which our health depends. The earth element is placed in the southwest of the plot or building.

AIR

Every organism needs air to survive, plants and animals are now inducing human mutually dependent upon each other for their survival; animals need the respired oxygen from plants, and plants need the carbon dioxide that animals respire. All living organism are in balance with the oceans and atmosphere and Gaia maintains this equilibrium with astounding accuracy.

Air Pollution

The air pollution is positively affecting every living organism.

Natural Air Pollution

Nature pollutes the air in many ways without our help. Sulphur oxides and particulates from forest fires and volcanoes, dust from wind storms, the hydrocarbons and pollens of plants that live on the methane and the hydrogen sulphide given off by decaying vegetation, viruses and dust from soil, the salt particulate carbon monoxide, carbon dioxide and oxides of nitrogen all result in various degrees of air pollution.

Human Air Pollution

The atmosphere is a gift from nature, which costs us nothing and requires only care for its quality. Humanity generates pollutants in such concentrations that this ultimate environmental amenity may become the ultimate environmental obscenity.

The major primary human air pollutants are carbon monoxide, sulphur oxides, oxides of nitrogen, lead, hydrocarbons, photochemical oxidants particulate and radiation.

Indoor Air Pollution

In the United States, the Environmental Protection Agency has identified 1000 pollutants that occur indoors, 60 of which can cause cancer. The building of healthy houses, free from indoor Pollution and causing as little damage to the atmosphere as possible, is paramount to maintaining the health of occupants and the balance of life on this planet. The air element is placed in the north-west of the plot or building.

WATER

Every drop of water has been here since the beginning of the earth. Water circulates in complex pathways and therefore needs to be conserved and its purity protected. Some 97 percent of all water is sea water which covers three- quarters of the Earth's surface. Of the remaining 3 percent, 2.94 percent is captured in the ice caps and at inaccessible depths in the earth. This leaves only 0.06 percent of all the water in the world as usable fresh water.

Contaminated Water

Throughout the world water is being contaminated in a variety of ways, diminishing the amount of fresh, healthy water available.

Disease

Water, the ultimate sustaining element of life, kills some 25 million people in developing nations each year. Sixty percent of these are children. Their scarce water supplies are used over and over, becoming a breeding ground for pathogens and disease carriers, resulting in outbreaks of diarrheas infections, dysentery, salmonella, typhoid and cholera. The situation is made worse by the dumping of waste products in rivers and oceans.

SPACE

Space is the sea of radiation and energy which creates the necessary conditions for the life, health and demise of all organisms. It could be said to embrace the geo-energetic, electromagnetic, electrostatic and gravitational forces exerted upon us by the Earth, the sun and other planets. It is the universal substance, the vital essence known as akasha in the Hindu Vedas. The space element is placed in the centre of the plot or building.

3

Factors Affecting Sick Building Syndrome

Sun and Seasonal Affective Disorder

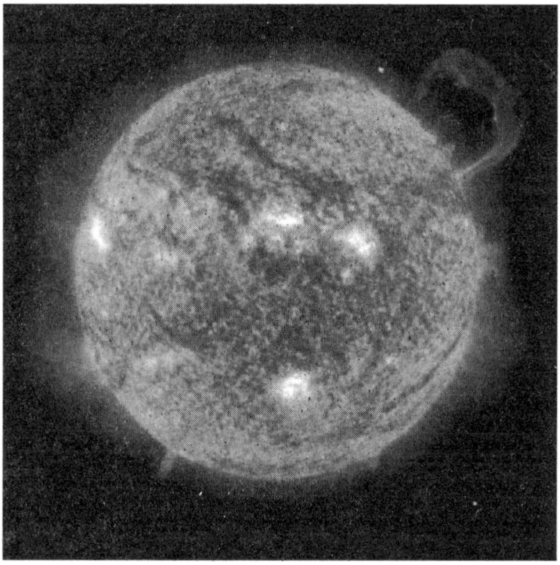

The Sun

It is believed that the Sun was formed about five billion years ago from a rotating mass of gas and dust. Due to compressed it gradually warmed up to temperatures of 15 million degrees. At this point nuclear fusion began in its core, and energy in the form of heat and light travelled out from the centre.

The sun is composed of 74 percent hydrogen, 25 percent helium, and 1 percent other elements, more than sixty of which are naturally occurring elements of Earth. The Sun is about 150 million kilometres from the Earth. Its diameter is around 1.4 million kilometres. The temperature at the core of the Sun is approximately 15 million degrees Celsius. The coolest part of the Sun is nearly 6,000 degrees Celsius.

The Sun has a strong magnetic field like a bar magnet in some aspects. But this magnetic field is irregular due to the movement of gases whose atoms are ionized. Particles trapped in a magnetic field usually follow the magnetic lines of force but the motion of large quantities of plasma tends to change the direction of these lines. It is this change in the pattern that gives rise to the Sun's activities.

Sun gives us Heat, Light and Energy

Light from the Sun is the natural source of light that heats the Earth and makes life on Earth possible. Humans, animals & Plants all need sunlight to grow. Our life completely depends on the Sun or else there is a lifeless life without sun.

Sunlight is made of tiny units of radiant energy called photons. The Photons are born in the centre of the Sun's core. Each photon carries a speck of energy and trillions of photons hit each square meter of Earth every second. A group of photons are called sunlight. Clouds, water and ground, all reflect sunlight in the space and makes earth visible from a spaceship. The amount of energy that is carried by the wave of light or a photon largely determines the colour of the light.

Light is an electromagnetic wave as it consists of both electric as well as magnetic fields. The electromagnetic radiations from sun exist in different wavelengths. The red wavelengths of the light are called long waves while violet wavelengths are called short waves. All the other colours lie between these long and short waves. Colours in the nature exist or are seen because of sunlight. Therefore the total world of beauty and aesthetics exist because of sunlight.

Energy from the Sun sets the Earth's weather in motion. Heat from the Sun causes water on the Earth's surface to evaporate and form clouds that eventually provide fresh rainwater. Winds occur because the Sun's rays are more direct and thus stronger at the equator than they are at poles. The strong rays in tropical regions warm the air there, causing it to rise. Cool air from the polar regions then flows under the warm tropical air. These movements create air currents that circulate around the Earth. These are influenced by the Earth's rotation, the surface features of the continents and variations in the amount of moisture in the atmosphere.

Sunlight and Health

Sunlight has a deep relationship with health. It was known in the past too, that sunlight striking the skin initiated a series of reaction in the body leading to the production of Vitamin D, a necessary ingredient for the absorption of calcium and other minerals from the diet. If Vitamin D is absent, the body will not absorb the amount of calcium required for normal growth and development of bones.

The cosmic cycles affect our universe, which then affects the Solar System, which then affects the Earth and so on down through Earth's Climate, season's inhabitants, right down to the smallest particle within an atom. Since all things are integrally connected in this way, everything affects everything else. Nothing escapes this process.

Sun Light–Sustainer of Healthy Life

Energy from Sunlight

1. The Sun is the abundant rechargeable energy to make life comfortable and to prosper on this planet EARTH.
2. Energy from the nature is the base of Vastu Science. The whole universe is a dynamic Web of inspire able energy pattern, the solar energy and the earth energy. Duration of time study for exhausting of Earth energy resources.
3. Human beings get maximum energy from sun which is rhythm of daily life in form of warmth and light for all actions / reactions for all the life form of Universe. A Vastu Consultant and Architect should learn to balance the natural energies, especially the Sun in design process so as to produce an environment full of energy.

Life on Earth is under the constant influence of natural Sunlight. World have always recognized connection with sun light. It was profoundly recognized by the ancient cultures that they revered the sun as God for its blessing. Since sunlight containing Ultra Violet Rays (Invisible form of light) is beneficial to humans, and there are certain adverse effects too. Let us not say that the God may have made mistake in giving harmful Ultra Violet light & Rays

In the Vedic period, people built homes, temples, and hermitages, applying Vastu principle, by balancing the five elements with a view to have a peaceful living, offering prayers and to live in common harmony. But in the modern world people built concrete clusters, mainly for a high rate of return. After the second world war, the architectural practice has turned into a race towards the so-called Modernization. Adopting bureaucratic values, that have resulted in worldwide pollution, environmental and ecological problems; with no peace of mind whatsoever, under any kind of shelter.

What are Ultra Violet Rays?

Ultraviolet rays are an invisible form of light. They lie just beyond the violet end of the visible spectrum. The sun is the major nature source of ultraviolet rays. Lightning, or any other electrical spark in the air, also emits ultraviolet rays. The rays can be produced artificially by passing an electric current through a gas or vapour, such as mercury vapour. Ultraviolet rays can cause sunburn. Overexposure to these rays can cause skin cancer. Ultraviolet rays also destroy harmful organisms and have other useful effects.

Ultraviolet rays have shorter wavelengths than visible light has. A wavelength the distance between the crests of two waves, is often measured in units called nanometers One nanometers (NM) equals 0.000001 millimeter (0.000000039 inch.) wavelength of visible light range from about 400 to 700 nm. Ultraviolet wavelength range from about 1 to 400 nm. The wavelength of Ultra violet rays determines whether a material they shine on absorbs the rays or transmits them. For example, only ultra violet rays with shorter wavelengths can pass through ordinary window glass. The glass absorbs rays with shorter wavelength, though they can pass through other materials.

Ultra Violet Light

Ultra Violet Light is an effective treatment for many diseases. The sun therapy is very commonly used as Naturopathy Therapy included treatment of anameia, gouts, colities, cystities, arteriosclerosis, rheumatoid arthiritis, eczema, acne, herpes, lupus, sciatica, asthma, kidney problems and even burns. People will have to understand that there are lot of health benefits from ultraviolet light as enumerated below:-

1. UV Light increases the efficiency of heart. At the Tulane School of Medicine, Dr. Raymond Johnson exposed 20 people to Ultra Violet Light. In 18 of out of the 20 people their cardiac out put increased an average of 39% ! In other words, their hearts became stronger and pumped more blood.
2. UV Light reduces cholesterol. In one experiment, patients with hypertension and related circulatory problems were exposed to UV Light. Two hours after the first exposure, 97% of the patients had almost a 13% decrease in serum Cholesterol levels.
3. UV Light is an effective treatment for psoriasis. Reports from the National Psoriasis Foundation indicate that 80% of those suffering from this skin disease improve when they are exposed to U V Light.
4. UV Light activates the synthesis of Vitamin D, which is a prerequisite for the absorption of calcium and other minerals from the diet. Robert Neer and Associates conducted a study on a group of elderly persons to determine if extra sunlight would increase their ability to absorb calcium from their diets. The group which did not receive UV rays had 25% decrease in Calcium absorption while the other group receiving UV Rays had a 15% increase in absorption.
5. UV Light increases the level of sex hormones. In a study at Boston State Hospital, Dr. Abraham Myerson found that ultra violet light increased

male hormones level by 120%. UV Light activates an important skin hormone.

6. UV Light is an effective treatment for many diseases indicated above. UV Light has been found very effective in killing infectious bacteria, including several forms of tuberculosis bacteria.

Today, practically all sources of ultra violet exposure are seen as detrimental to humans. It is well known that tuberculosis was one of the main disease that was treated by Sunlight and many patients were completely cured. It is very important to know & study in deep the U V Light and Infra Red Rays, but first we must know that too much UV light is bad, "we need a basic amount to support life and maintain a healthy immune system." If someone says that oxygen is hazardous to our health we will say he does not understand gift of nature. Similar is conclusion for Ultra violet light. People are spending most of their lives under artificial lighting and suffering. They have to understand about advantage and disadvantage of Ultra Violet light.

Since sunlight (containing UV) is beneficial to humans and that there are certain adverse effects to persons living and working in artificial lighting. The light in most houses looks yellowish and dingy. The wavelengths of light in the orange – pink – red range caused laboratory animals to lose their hair, show excessive calcium deposits in their hearts and develop large fast growing tumors. He also found that when animals cells were exposed to red and infra red portions of the spectrum, their cell walls ruptured and cell division process (mitosis) stopped. Sunlight consists of a fairly balanced spectrum of color. Interestingly enough, blue is the wavelength most lacking in incandescent light bulbs. It has been established that ultraviolet light is a nutrient, just like a vitamin or a mineral. Daily allowance for U V light has, therefore, recommended just as incase of vitamin C.

In fact overexposure to the sun, in conjunction with certain skin types, is a major factor in the development of skin cancer. The solution is quite simple, mild, sensible exposure to sunlight is not only safe, it is desirable. One of the constituent of sun light is "ultra-voilet" (UV) rays for which modern science has made us to think that it causes cancer, cataracts, aging and wrinkles. This blocking of ultra Violet rays may severely weaken the body's defenses. According to photo biologist Dr. john Ott, there are strong indications that UV light through eyes stimulates the immune system. UV light in large amount is harmful ; however in trace amounts, UV rays in nature sunlight, it acts, as a "life-supporting nutrient " which is highly beneficial. Sunlight contains different ultraviolet (UV) radiation. UV light is classified as UV-A, UV-B, or UV-C depending on its wavelength. UV-A (320-380 NM), directly adjoining the violet end of the visible-light spectrum is responsible for the tanning response in humans. UV-B (290-320 NM) activates the synthesis of vitamin D and the absorption of calcium and other minerals. UV-C (100-290 NM).

Uses of Ultra Violet Rays

Ultra violet rays with wavelength shorter than 300 nm are effective in killing bacteria and viruses. Hospitals use germicidal lamps that produce these short rays to sterilize surgical instruments, water and the air in operating rooms. Many food and drug companies use germicidal lamps to disinfect various types of products and their containers. Direct exposure to ultra violet rays with wavelengths shorter than 320 nm produces vitamin D in the body. Physicians once used sun lamps that produced these rays to prevent and treat rickets, a bone diseases caused by the lack of Vitamin D. The lamps are used today to treat some skin disorders, such acne and psoriasis. Some instruments use ultra violet rays to identify the chemical composition of unknown materials. Medical researchers use such instruments to analyze substances in the human body, including amino acids, enzymes, and other proteins. The electronics industry uses ultraviolet rays in manufacturing integrated circuits.

Harmful effects–The Sun's shortest ultraviolet rays those with wavelength below about 320 nm are particularly harmful to living things. Too much exposure to these rays can cause painful eye irritation or eye inflammation. High quality sun glasses protect the eyes from these rays. Over exposure to ultra violet rays also can cause a painful burn. Melanin, a brown pigment in the skin, provides some protection against sunburn. Sunscreen lotion absorbs the sun's burning rays.

Exposure to the sun ultra violet rays over a long period can cause skin cancer and other changes in human cells. Such exposure also can damage or kill plants. Ozone a form of oxygen in earth's upper atmosphere, absorbs most of the sun's ultra violet radiation. Without the ozone layer, ultra violet rays would probably destroy most plant and animal life.

Scientific Research–Ultra violet rays originate within the atoms of the elements. Scientists learn about the makeup and energy levels of atoms by studying the rays. Experts also learn about distant stars and galaxies by analyzing the ultra violet rays that they give off.

Much research has focused on the role of ultra violet rays in chemical reactions that break down the earth's protective ozone layer. As the ozone layer breaks down it becomes less effective as a barrier against harmful ultra violet rays. Experiments indicate that bees, butterflies, and other insects can see ultra violet light. The reflection of ultra violet rays off wings reveals patterns that help insects identify mates.

What are Infra Red Rays

The sun ultra violet rays struck or fall on any object or human beings etc. on the Earth, produce Infra red in relation to its temperature then surrounding temperature.

Infra red rays are often called heat rays, resemble light rays, but they cannot be seen by the human eye. They behave similarly to light rays in both Reflection and Refraction. Any object such as building material, metal furniture and much more made out of conductor and less in insulation etc. gives, off infra red rays in relation to its temperature. As an object gets hotter, it gives off more and more infra red rays. Such devices as the sniperscope, which was invented during world war II (1939-1945), can pick up infrared rays from object that are warmer than their surroundings. In this way, these devices can "see" such objects in the dark or through fog.

Photographers use film that is sensitive to infrared rays to take pictures in places where there is no visible light. Doctors use infrared lamps to treat skin diseases and sore muscles. In these treatments, the infrared rays pass through the patient's skin and produce heat when they strike the affected area.

Infrared waves lie just beyond the red end of the visible light spectrum. Sir William Herschel, a British astronomer, discovered infrared rays in 1800 by observing the effect of the heat they produced.

How to use Sun Rays for a Good Health?

With the previous explanation we come to a conclusion that U/V rays with W / L 1 to 300 n. m. is harmful for human consumption and W / L of 320 n.m. produces Vitamin D in our body and about 320 to 400 is good for human consumption. Now the early morning sun rays reaches the Earth Surface, passes through Ozone with more area, though reaches the earth surface with lesser radiation and cover more earth surface. Though the W/L during sun rise up to 2 hrs. is 320 to 400 nm is good for human consumption and if it mixes with cold water it multiplies the vitamin capacity and is very good for human skin & eye as well as produces positive energy. As sun rises it comes closer to the earth and distance of W/L between the crust comes closer much below 300 nm & between 10 :00 a.m. to 4:00 p.m. becomes Infra Red Ray's.

Solar Architecture and Energy Conservation through Building Design

Today, the world finds itself in the grip of an energy crisis more particular in 21st century. Known sources of conventional energy are dwindling very fast. The demand for energy especially in the third world is growing. And their efforts for development are constantly being threatened by environmental issues. The developed nations, who are the largest consumers and producers of energy, find themselves threatened by the potential energy, find themselves threatened by the potential energy crunch.

This has aroused an interest in the development of energy resources as well as conservation of the available sources. And a lot of research and thinking is being generated in this new field. Solar energy, bio-technology and superconductivity have the highest priorities in research fields. We, in India, have very low energy consumption levels as compared to the level of the consumption in developed countries. However much we may wise to increase the production of conventional energy, our efforts are going to face resistance. Narmada project is a very good example of this. Hence before achieving any increase in the consumption of energy, we have to start thinking of conserving the same.

This situation forces upon us the issues of conservation of energy techniques. We can learn from the developed nation's efforts in this sphere. It gives us a chance to reallocate our resources in better ways even before the energy situation becomes acute. Building construction, building design and architecture are such fields where the studies and research in energy conservation and renewable energy can be applied innovatively and creatively. Passive solar energy system collect transport heat by natural means. Passive system are simple in concept and use. The most striking difference between passive and active system is that the former operates on the energy available in its immediate environment and the latter imports energy to make the system work.

Solar Control

The age-old problems of controlling the reception of solar radiation in buildings have been sharply enlarged by the modern developments in architectural planning and construction. Traditional massive bearing-walls, which combined the function of support with protection from light and heat, have been supplanted by clear structural members devoted to load- bearing (the skeleton) and covered with curtain walls (the skin) made of many materials.

The skin of a building performs the role of a filter between indoor and outdoor conditions, to control the intake of air, heat, cold, light, sounds, and odors. It is generally agreed that air, temperature, wind, and sound are best controlled within the wall itself, while light is easier to control inside the building shell, and heat radiation is most efficiently halted before it reaches the building envelope proper.

The materials of a building skin play a decisive part in the utilization and control of solar rays. The first example is a full glass window wall. With its straight approach, appealing as it is, the wall has to absorb all the penalties of the environmental variations, since the bare glass pane offers very little (around 12%) protection from radiation.

The selective absorptivity and emissivity characteristics of materials are another very effective defense against radiation impacts and especially important in over-heated conditions. Materials which reflect rather than absorb radiation and which more readily release the absorbed quantity as thermal radiation, will cause lower temperatures with in the structure. The sun's energy, by the time it falls upon a building, has been cut down by the atmosphere and arrives through several through several different channels. The solar radiation consists of visible wavelengths (0.3 to 0.7 microns). Since this energy is concentrated near the visible part of the spectrum, the criterion of reflectivity is an approximate relation to color values. White materials may reflect 90% or more, black materials 15% or less, of the radiation received.

On the other hand, the thermal exchange with the surroundings consists of longer infrared wavelengths (over 2.5 usually from 5 to 20 microns. This range can also be classified as 9 microns. The characteristics of materials in regards to reflectivity of long - wave infrared heat depend more on the density of surface and on molecular composition than on color. The summer rays of high elevation may be intercepted by building elements of high reflectivity. In zones where hot conditions prevail, the net effect of reflectivity combined with the emissive thermal radiation characteristic of the material has to be considered.

If surfaces exposed to the irradiation of the sun and to a clear sky are whitewashed, painted white or built of light-colored material such as marble, they will remain cooler than surface of polished metal such as aluminum. Despite the fact that aluminum has a higher reflectivity to solar radiation, the effect is outbalanced by the emissive capability of the white surface which loses heat by thermal radiation toward the sky. This principle accounts for the white exteriors of tropical buildings. However, if the same materials are exposed not only to the sun but to hot ground where the white surface is hot capable are losing heat by emissivity, the polished aluminum will be the cooler of the two materials. The application of both processes is utilized by aeroplanes, where the upper part exposed to solar radiation is painted white, while the lower portion remains metallic. By converting solar energy into heat, heating can be provided locally.

Sun and Health

An adequate level of sunlight can positively alter the mood chemically and even prevent depression. SAD Seasonal Affective Disorder is a mood disorder in which people experience depressive symptoms due to lack of adequate levels of sunlight especially winters. SAD was first formally described and named in 1984 by Norman E. Rosenthal and at the National

Institute of Mental Health. The US National Library of Medicine states that "some people experience a serious mood change when the seasons change. They may sleep too much, have little energy, and may also feel depressed. Though symptoms can be severe, they usually clear up. The condition in the summer is often referred to as reverse seasonal affective disorder, and can also include heightened anxiety".

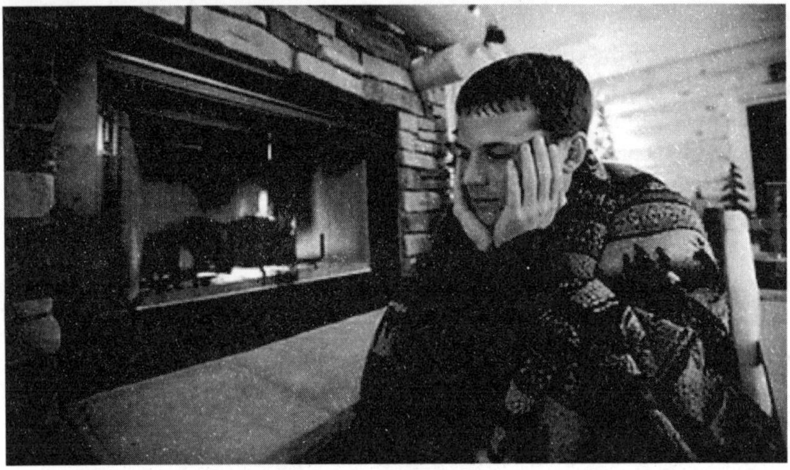

Seasonal Affective Disorder

Symptoms of Winter SAD–

- Lack of Energy
- Difficulty in Concentration
- Lack of Socialisation
- Depression
- Pessimistic Feelings of Hopelessness
- Lack of Pleasure
- Morning Sickness
- Craving for Carbohydrates
- Sudden Weight Gain
- Craving for Sweets
- Tendency to Oversleep
- Tendency to Overeat
- Craving for Carbohydrates, which leads to weight-gain and may characterize the presence of disorder

Symptoms of Summer SAD–

- Depression
- Insomnia
- Anxiety
- Irritability
- Decreased Appetite
- Intense Sadness
- Weight Loss
- Social Withdrawal
- Increased Sex Drive

The one and only cause of seasonal affective disorder is lack of natural sunlight on skin. When one does not receive enough natural sunlight one may suffer from a nutritional deficiency. It can also be referred as "sunlight deficiency".

Hibernation is an extreme example of sunlight deficiency but even species that do not hibernate often exhibit changes in behaviour during the winter. It has been argued that SAD is an evolved adaptation in humans that is a variant or remnant of a hibernation response in some remote ancestor.

If a person makes a point to get natural sunlight on their skin on a frequent basis daily,it is certain that person will experience a wide range of healthful benefits, including improvement in mood and an ending of any state of depression they may have experienced, increased bone density and reversal of symptoms of osteoporosis, help in reversing prostate cancer and breast cancer, and enhanced mood and brain function.

A Harvard study published in the January 13 issue of the respected medical journal, Neurology " the scientific journal of the American Academy of Neurology " has identified a lack of Vitamin D as a principle indicator in incidence of the deadly, debilitating disease, multiple sclerosis in women. In addition, sunshine may protect against the development of multiple sclerosis, according to the findings of an Oxford University study to be published in next month's Journal of Epidemiology and Community Health.

Earlier research also points to the role of vitamin D in MS. In MS patients, levels of Vitamin D in the body can predict periods of low or high disease activity " the higher the Vitamin D, the lower the disease activity. Scientists believe that the hormone Serotonin is responsible for SAD and affects the sleep, eating behaviours, and mood regulation.

Sunlight also stimulates the pineal gland - a tiny pea-sized organ found in the base of the brain. It is also referred to as 'the third eye', the pineal gland produces certain types of brain chemicals called 'tryptamines'. One type of tryptamine, melatonin, keeps our body clock aware of day and night, and the changing seasons. From the spiritual perspectives, sunlight helps an individual to raise all the levels of consciousness within including simple consciousness, self consciousness and cosmic consciousness. It is considered to be the life force and best healer in the nature. Sun has always been considered as the God of health. The light of the sun has been used by healers for healing various diseases.

Experts suggest that the influence of Sunlight may be related to the number of red cells and haemoglobin in the blood. An insufficiency of light may cause an increase in the serum or watery portion of the blood and a corresponding decrease in the quantity of blood fibrin and red corpuscles, resulting in anemia. Sunlight may also favorably influence the irregularities of ovulation, pubertal difficulties and impotency. Studies have shown that after prolonged fasting or a wasting illness, exposure to sufficient Sunshine may enable the body to gain energy.

Scientists today also believe that sunlight may reduce the risk of several types of cancer such as breast, colon, ovary, bladder, womb, stomach and prostate gland.

Diseases and Sunlight

Vitamin D

The Sun plays a very important role in the formation of vitamin D in our body. When Sunlight penetrates our skin, vitamin D is produced. Vitamin D is called the 'Sunshine vitamin' because it is formed in the skin when the body is exposed to Sunlight. This vitamin is essential for our health. A major source of this vitamin is produced through the interaction of the Sun with certain chemicals in our body.

Vitamin D is essential for calcium and phosphorous metabolism in our body. It helps prevent rickets. The deficiency as well as the excess of this vitamin can seriously affect the bones. Ten minutes of daily exposure to sunlight can supply us with all the vitamin D that we need. Recent laboratory experiments suggest that vitamin D can also prevent the growth and spread of cancerous tumours.

Bones

Sunlight is vital for proper bone development. Calcium and phosphorous help in transformation of cartilage into bone. When there is insufficient exposure to sunlight, then defective and brittle bones may result. Sunlight helps in the assimilation of calcium and because of that it is of great value in the prevention of rickets and tuberculosis. A lack of calcium is associated with both these conditions.

Skin

Sun helps in maintaining good skin and acts like a natural disinfectant for the body. Tanning is skin's natural response to UV light. It is a reaction, just like an allergic reaction, to prevent further injury to skin from the Sun. Too much Sunlight can be harmful; it can burn the skin especially in hot and humid weather. Sunburns can be mild and severe. The skin turns red in mild Sunburn and the redness disappears in a few days. But repeated Sun tanning may also contribute to skin cancer and wrinkling.

Heat Stroke

Heat stroke is one of the most common yet deadly effects of the Sun on the body. A heat stroke results because of a serious failure of the body's heat regulation mechanisms due to excessive exposure to intense heat.

Heat Exhaustion

Many a times when you feel the heat and you sweat a lot, you feel the exhaustion or get that tired feeling and feel giddy. Other signs of heat exhaustion include nausea, headaches, moist clammy skin, and pale or flushed skin. Heat exhaustion is caused by a loss of fluid through sweating. Severe heat exhaustion can result in unconsciousness and the person would require medical treatment.

Heat Cramps and Fainting

When one works continuously in heat or in the Sun, one may suffer from heat cramps or fainting. The cramps are painful spasms of the muscles. One can treat heat cramps by drinking liquids in moderate amounts. Fainting is again a common problem. Lay down the person who feels like fainting. Movement will prevent people from fainting.

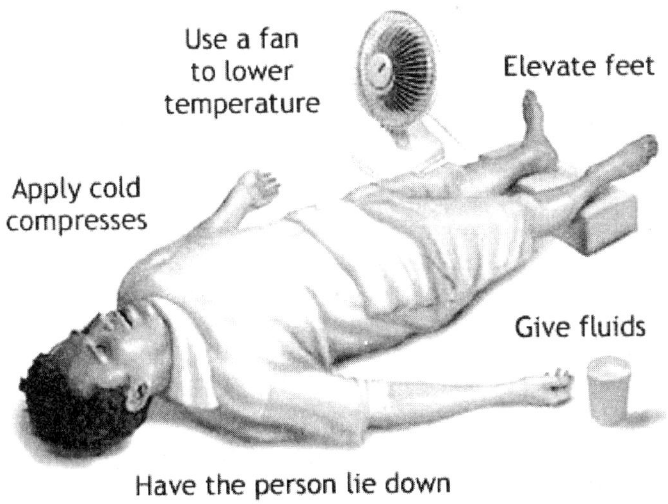

Fainting

Multiple Sclerosis

MS is influenced by multiple interacting genetic, environmental, nutritional, hormonal, immunological, and viral factors. It is strongly correlated with sunlight, which is a function of latitude, season, prevailing weather, etc. People with MS are often vitamin-D deficient. Recently, Harvard University investigators examined data collected from two long-term studies involving 187,000 women. The data indicated that those who consumed the most vitamin D had a substantially lower MS risk than women who consumed the least amount. Many scientists believe that vitamin D mediates its healing influence by interacting with MS's dysfunctional immune system. Vitamin D profoundly influences the expression of 1) a variety of immune cells, which possess gene-modulating, vitamin-D receptors, and 2) key immune-mediating molecules called *cytokines.*

Overall Health

Evidence indicates that vitamin D prevents cancer, diabetes, arthritis, high-blood pressure, cardiovascular disease, and infections. In other words, it enhances overall wellness. **Now days buildings do not receive adequate sunlight at adequate timings. Due to lack of sunlight, occupants suffer from Sick Building Syndrome.**

Solution to Seasonal Affective Disorder

Lack of Sunlight is the problem whereby receiving adequate levels of sunlight is the solution. Everybody needs to expose their skin to natural sunlight for limited time without using sunscreen for a few minutes each day. In case if an apartment does not receive enough sunlight, the occupants should either go to the terrace or to a neighbouring park to receive sunlight. Exercise can be helpful. The occupants should prefer warm colours inside and outside the building. The tints and shades of red, orange and yellow should be preferred. The occupants should also use warm light (tungsten bulb) inside.

A balanced diet comprising more vegetables, fruits, and complex carbohydrates will also help. Sugars, processed or junk foods should be avoided. As SAD is a psychological disorder and may require professional medical diagnosis and treatment. Spectrometry can also be of utmost help in healing SAD.

Extreme Climatic Conditions and Sick Building Syndrome

Climatic Planning and Designing

The energy requirement of a building depends upon various factors like comfort requirements location of building, usage of building etc.

Climatology and its effect on Men–Building and Building Material

Man's energy and health depend in large measures on the direct effects of his environment. It is well known that in certain climatic areas, where excessive heat or cold prevails, energy is eliminated by the biological strain of adaptation to the extreme conditions. Physical and psychological strains

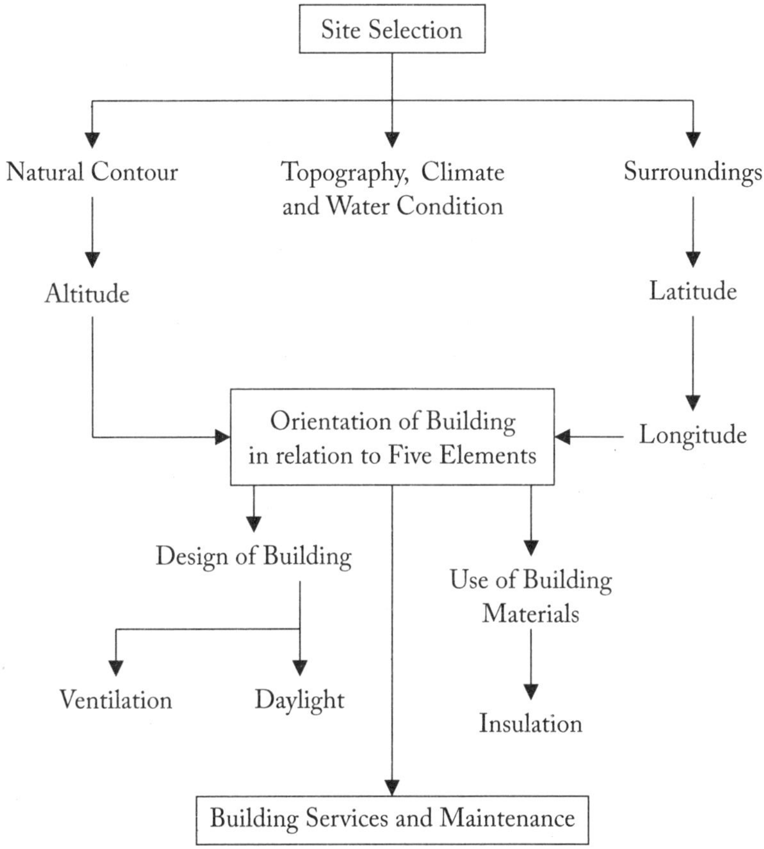

result from this struggle for biological equilibrium. The design, which in a given environment setting reduces undesirable stress, and at the same time utilizes all natural resources favourable to human living comfort would be considered responsive to climate.

In Vedic Period, Vastu Shastra suggested that the environment to be made livable by careful selection and orientation of building, including placement of opening, thermal efficiency of building materials, layout and space planning according to the solar and wind conditions, shading devices, vegetation and waterbodies. The Vastu consultant, therefore, had to remain alert to micro climatic conditions and regional variations. There are such examples of vernacular architectural in various climatic zones of India. Building industry consumes vast resources of energy through all phases of development, starting from the production of building materials, to its use and maintenance. Besides the scarcity, and their rising cost, their negative

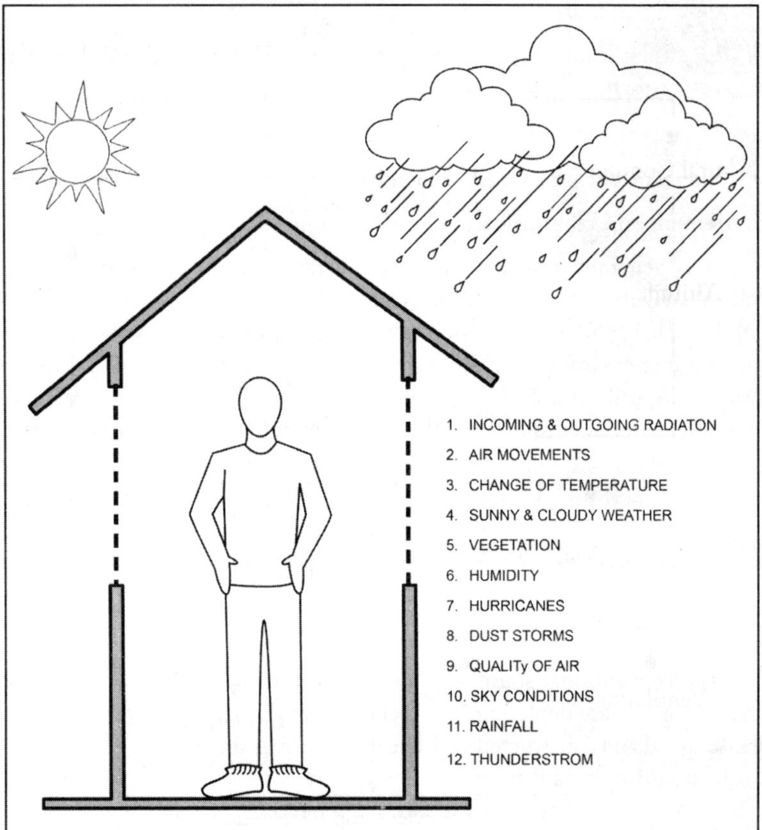

Micro Climate Affects Human Body

environmental impacts has shifted the emphasis from energy utilization to energy conservation. The need today in 21st century is to draw from the experiences of the past and blend it with the modern concepts and realities, in creating buildings, which are harmonious with the natural environment. The desirable procedure, to work towards such requirements would be to work with and not against the forces of nature.

Climatic Parameters

Climate	*Weather*	*Micro Weather*
Average weather over a period of many years.	Integration variable atmosphere for a period of time.	Integration variable Atmosphere for a brief particular place for a brief period of time.

These parameters are–

- Solar Radiation
- Air Humidity
- Air temperature
- Wind speed and direction
- Wind pressure
- Precipitation

These are the parameters, which have an effect on the building design.

Settlement and Habitation at Comfort Zone

It is generally agreed that air, temperature, wind and sound are best controlled within the wall itself, while light is easier to control inside the building shell, the heat radiation is most efficiently halted before it reaches the building environment. The materials of the building skin play a decisive part in the utilization and control of solar rays. The thermal efficiency of different material accounts for the variation in indoor climate with similar building skins. A good understanding of the thermal behavior of building materials is essential for any energy efficient planning. The total problem of orientation for buildings other than the thermal Consists of optimization factors like the habits of people living in a particular topography which are an important indicator of how they have been facing the vagaries of nature.

Climatic Efficient Building Design

The conventional sources of energy are rather limited and the present known sources are depleting fast. Generally, at the planning stages buildings are designed and constructed with the initial cost as the primary consideration. Little attention is paid to ensure low energy consumption. Efficient energy management is the need of the day. New buildings should be planned and existing modified to reduce the energy requirements to the optimum levels. Vernacular architecture in various climatic zones of India such as in Udaipur, Jaipur, Sansad Bhawan- Delhi with shaded balcony corridor around show how optimization has been achieved.

In 21st century, modern building industry with its significant achievements in housing is providing comforts to a growing population; unfortunately it is highly dependent upon the easy availability of energy. Building industry consumes vast resources of energy through all phases of development, starting from the production of building materials, to its use and maintenance. In view of recent energy crisis all over the world, importance of utilization of solar energy and other natural means of heating and cooling of buildings are being explored and adopted. The solar passive systems have been used and tested with encouraging results.

Climate and Humans

Climate of a region affects living beings directly and indirectly. Changes in temperature are directly felt and human adapts himself by wearing clothes appropriate to the season. Woollen clothes worn in winter protect us from cold. Cotton clothes are preferred in the hot summer as they absorb sweat and allow air circulation. People living in colder regions use tight fitting clothes, while those living in tropical regions wear loose garments, which permit movement of air so that the body is kept cool. Exposure to extremes of temperature during heat waves or cold waves may cause death. Climatic changes resulting in droughts and floods affect man directly. Climatic conditions may have a direct affect on the physical & mental condition of a occupant. For example too much of cold winds from north direction in hilly areas can be extremely bad for the health of occupants. It is essential to create comfortable conditions inside, merge with the climatic conditions existing and leave the extreme conditions outside the building.

Houses built by humans are also adapted to the climatic conditions. In India, for example, in regions of heavy rainfall like Kerala, & the North East state of Assam, houses have steeply sloping roofs to drain off the rainwater. Flat roofs are commonly found in desserts. In cooler regions, houses have glass panels for doors and windows to allow more sunlight and heat. In warmer regions, houses have broad verandahs to protect them from direct sunlight. Windows are large to allow greater circulation of air so that the inside of the house remains cooler than the outside. In mountain regions like the Himalayas, South-facing slopes are preferred for construction of houses as they are exposed to sunlight. Humans are now using mechanical devices like fans, air-conditioners, heaters, humidifiers etc, to overcome adverse climatic conditions and to live in comfort. Such devices however consume large quantities of energy.

Study of Local environment

The local environment around a place may be studied by making field trips. Observations may be made about the landforms, rivers, source of water supply, drainage, land-use, crops cultivated etc, covering both natural environment and cultural aspects. Examples of environmental pollution may also be noted.

Weather–Weather is our most common topic of conversation. Hardly a day passes without weather-phenomenon claiming headlines in newspapers of news broadcasts. These may include reports of heavy floods causing breach and damage, with considerable loss of life and prosperity, in squalls or hail storms or lighting strikes.

Meteorology–It is the branch of science, which deals with the earth's atmosphere and the physical processes in it. It includes the study of the changing atmospheric conditions- such as rain, wind thunder storm, snow, fog, which go to make up our weather. Meteorology is comparatively a young science. Meteorologist attempt to forecast future weather over a place or region on the basis of a large number of actual weather observations recorded at fixed time at meteorological observations.

Value of Weather Knowledge

Weather plays an important part in all aspects of human life, be it personal, social or economic. It is thus an inescapable phenomenon in human life. Weather plays vital and intimate role in architecture. It is the only knowledge of the weather elements that can enable Vastu advisor to design with maximum efficiency and comfort.

Atmosphere–The atmosphere is the shallow skin or envelope of gases surrounding the surface of the earth. If the earth is compared to a baseball, the atmosphere's thickness of the gaseous envelope or skin is still a matter of argument. What is known is that there is no sharp limit to it, and is, somewhere between 200 and 600 miles up.

Composition of Air–Although extremely light, air has weight and is highly elastic and compressible. It is a mixture of gases, of many gases entering into its composition, chief are Nitrogen (comprising 78% of the volume of the dry air) and Oxygen (comprising 21%), Argon, Carbondioxide, Hydrogen, neon, Helium, Krypton and Xenon are also present in very small quantities. Besides these fixed components, the atmosphere also contains water vapour in variable amounts.

Air envelopes the entire surface of earth on which we live. Although it is not visible to us we can always feel it. When we run fast, it opposes our motion and when it is in fast motion, it can uproot even big trees. The fast moving air is called storm. Air is absolutely essential for life. No living and being plant or animal can survive without it. It gives us energy and plants get their food from the carbon dioxide present in it. Water vapour in the air helps to produce rains. The quantity of water vapour in the air varies from place to place. The desert air is dry whereas the air in the areas adjoining the sea contains considerable amount of water vapour. This is why it rains heavily in places near the sea.

Presence of Water Vapour–Although an invisible gas, water vapour is a very important constituent of the atmosphere, under certain conditions water vapour can condense into the millions of tiny droplets of water or crystals of ice which constitutes fog near the frond and clouds. Clouds produce rain, snow or thunderstorm and also prevent partially, radiation of heat from the earth. It is therefore necessary to know something about the water vapour in the atmosphere, which produces weather.

Humidity and Saturation–The amount of water vapour in the air is called humidity. There is a limit to water vapour content of the air at any temperature.

Air at a given temperature in contact with a flat surface of pure water (or ice) can take only a limited amount of water vapour. The higher the temperature, the more water vapour it can contain. Air is said to be saturated at a particular temperature when it contains the maximum possible quantity of water vapour.

Relative Humidity–Relative humidity is a term used to express the degree of saturation of air. It is the percentage ratio of the amount of water vapour actually present in the air to the amount, which would be needed to saturate it at that temperature. When air can hold more water than it is cold. When the air with a given amount water vapour is warmed, its relative humidity decreases. If it is cooled, the relative humidity goes up. Normally the relative humidity of the air is highest at the time of the sunrise when the surface temperature is minimum and decreases as the temperature goes up.

Now the question comes, what is the source of moisture in the air? Moisture is always present in the air in the form of water vapour, but we are unable to see it. The amount of water vapour present in the air varies from place to place. Even the air in the big deserts contains some amount of water vapour. As we know, about 70% of the earth's surface is covered with water. Due to the solar heating water from the seas, rivers, lakes and ponds evaporate and mix with air. And thus the constant supply of water vapour to the air is maintained. In the scientific language the water vapour present in the air is called humidity. It varies from season to season. The amount of humidity is more during the summers than in winters. This is because large quantities of water from the seas, rivers, ponds etc gets converted into water vapour due to the higher atmospheric temperature during the summer. Also, the air expanded due to heating is capable of accommodating more water vapors. When it rains, the humidity increases tremendously, because a very large portion of the earth's surface is covered with water, which goes on evaporating into atmosphere.

It is the water vapour present in the air that causes the formation of the dew, fog, frost, snow etc. We get a lot of information about the weather by studying the variations in the humidity. The instrument, which measures humidity, is called 'Hygrometer'. High humidity indicates the possibility of rains. Cotton mills require humid atmosphere because the presence of moisture in the atmosphere prevents the breaking of cotton threads. Thus, we see that the study of humidity helps us in many ways.

Winds: Wind is defined as air in horizontal motion. Although the atmosphere has both horizontal and vertical motions of air, the horizontal motions have, in general, larger speeds, and their measurement both near the ground and at upper levels can be made with a much greater degree of accuracy than in the cause of vertical motions. Like any other fluid, air has got a natural tendency to move from a region of air surplus (high pressure) to one of air deficit (low pressure). This movement is the primary cause of wind. The speed of movement is proportional to the "gradient of pressure", i.e. the rate of change of pressure from high to low. Thus, if the pressure gradient were the only force, we would expect the wind to blow directly from high pressure to low pressure. It is the mixture of Oxygen, nitrogen, carbon dioxide, Water vapour and dust. Air in motion is called as wind.

When the sun's rays heat any place on the earth, the air of that place gets heated. Due to this heating, the air expands and hence its density decreases or it becomes lighter. The hot air, due to its lightness, goes up in the atmosphere. And this causes a decrease in atmosphere pressure in that area. Under such a condition air from high-pressure cool area rushes to that place to restore balance. This movement of air is called the 'blowing of the wind'. In the area adjoining the sea, the earth becomes hot during the day. Due to this, air becomes lighter and goes up in the atmosphere. To fill up the void so caused, cold air from the sea blows towards the land. During the night. A reverse movement takes place; that is, the earth becomes colder than the seawater and as such the air moves from the land towards the sea. It is very hot in the regions surrounding the equator. So there is a constant upward movement of hot air from these regions. The hot air flows out to the north and south. The rotation of the earth on its axis considerably effects the directions of the winds. The westerly winds are the direct result of the earth's rotation from west to east. The spinning of the earth makes all the winds in the Northern Hemisphere deflect towards the right and in the Southern Hemisphere towards the left. The presence of mountains also influences the wind direction. The mountains obstruct the winds and change their directions. The instrument used for measuring the wind velocity is called as 'Anemometer'.

Rain: Rain falls from clouds. Every cloud is made of water droplets or ice crystals. The growth of a cloud droplet to a size enough to fall out is the cause of the rain and other forms of precipitation. This important growth process is called coalescence. Coalescence occurs in following ways:

- Droplets in clouds are of different sizes. Big drops move more slowly in turbulent air and in path differ from the path of the small droplets. Bigger, heavier drops are not whipped around so rapidly. So drops collide, become bigger, and finally drop as rain. This is probably the main cause of rainfall from other low clouds.

- The most important type of coalescence occurs when tiny ice crystals and water droplets occur together (as near the middle of cumulonimbus clouds). Some water droplets evaporate and then condense on the crystals. The crystals grow until they drop as snow or ice pellets. As these drop through warm air, they change into raindrops.

- Lighting discharges in a thunderstorm form oxides of Nitrogen that are extremely hygroscope (water absorbing). These oxides are added to the atmosphere and become one of the kinds of nuclei for future condensation and eventual coalescence and rainfall. But the two processes mentioned above are the rain and perhaps the only causes of coalescence and hence precipitation. Research may show other possibilities.

Differences between Drizzle/Rain/Showers:

Drizzle – Fine drops diameter less than 0.5 mm.

Rain – Drops with diameter more than 0.5 mm.

Showers – Rain generally of short duration with sudden commencement.

The highest rainfall of the world takes place at Cherapunji (Assam) in India. The average annual rainfall of this place is 1200cms. In 1861, the total rainfall recorded here was 2175cms.

In summer, the wind blowing from the ocean towards the land spells the possibilities of rains whereas in winter blowing from the land towards the ocean is indicative of dryness. In south Asia, the wind from the Indian Ocean blowing towards the shore is the monsoon wind. This wind indicates the chances of rains. Monsoon is of two kinds: South Western or summer monsoon and North Eastern or winter monsoon. These winds advance from the Indian Ocean towards the shore in mid June and after being obstructed by the Himalayas cause rains in the plains. Contrary to this, in the winter, in the Central Asia and North India, very cold, dry and strong winds blow off shore. They are called winter monsoon or the retreating monsoon. They cause some rain in the coastal areas.

It is interesting to see how the monsoon winds change the coastal weather. It is a scientific truth that big sub-continents warm up or cool off much faster than the seas adjoining them. The areas of central and South Asia start warming up in the spring and by the summer become very hot in comparison to the India Ocean in the South and the Pacific Ocean in the east. Due to high temperature, there is a reduction in the air pressure on the land and consequently winds start blowing from the sea to the shore. This is the summer monsoon. With onset of autumn, the entire Asia starts cooling fast and by the winter, the temperature is much less than that of the adjoining oceans. This increases the atmospheric pressure and as such in the winter, monsoon winds start blowing from the dry shore to the seas. The South and East Asia have a monsoon climate because of their large landed area.

Microclimate and Macroclimate: The combined climatic conditions of a region small in area or the parts of a region characterize the microclimate are: temperature, humidity, means radiation temperature, velocity of air movement and level of light intensity and distribution. Microclimate is considerably affected by the terrain of the place (North or South slope, valley or upland), ground and soil conditions, plant life, the building pattern of the town, degree of air pollution, etc. The microclimate of an urban territory is thus regarded as the result of the interaction of natural and town planning factors such as water impounding, landscaping, asphalt paving, building density, etc.

Climate factors operate constantly throughout the year and hence the process of adaptation of people living, for example, in that tropics does not proceed in the same way as in regions with clearly defined seasons where the humans organism changes its protective properties to respond the changes in weather. We are inclined to think of the climate as certain uniformly distributed over a large area. This impression is partly because weather data are collected at points where "undisturbed conditions" prevail, and partly because large-scale maps depict equal mean temperatures in a few smooth lines. However, at ground level multifold minute climates exist side by side, varying sharply with the elevation of a few feet and within a distance of a mile. Plants are sensitive indicators of favorable circumstances. This effect is well known to farmers, who prefer southern slopes for growing grapes or cultivating orchards. Further, every elevation difference, character of land cover, every water surface, induces variations in a local climate. These effects within the large scale "macroclimate" form a small-scale pattern of "microclimates". Macro climate refers to climatic conditions of a larger area whereby microclimatic conditions apply to a site. Deviations in climate play an important part in architectural land utilization. First, in site selection, favorable locations should be considered. Second, a less favorable site may be improved by windbreaks and surrounding surfaces that induce an advantageous reaction to temperature and radiation impacts.

Human Life and Shelter: Mankind in the same environments encounters the same stresses as other fauna. Many scholars believed that climate had pronounced effects on human physiology and temperament. More recently interest has centered on human energy in relation to environment. Climate ranks with racial inheritance and cultural development as one of the apparently live in any region where he can obtain food, has strictly limited conditions under which his physical and mental energy (and even his moral character) can reach their highest development. The optimum climate conditions for human progress are:

1. Average temperature ranges from somewhat below 40 degrees F in the coldest months to nearly 70 degrees F in the warmest months.

2. Frequent storms or winds, to keep the relative humidity quiet high except in hot weather, and provide rain in all seasons.

3. A constant succession of cyclonic storms which bring frequent moderate changes in temperature but are not severe enough to be harmful.

The Effects of Climate on Man: Man's energy and health depend in large measure on the direct effects of his environment. It is a common experience to find that on some days the atmospheric conditions stimulate and invigorate our activities, while at other times they depress the physical and mental efforts. It is also well known that in certain climatic areas, where excessive heat or cold prevails, energy is diminished by the biological strain of adaptation to the extreme conditions.

The measurement of climatic effects has been investigated in many ways, here two methods of evaluation may be mentioned. One method describes the negative effects of climate on man, expressed as stress, pain, disease and death. The second defines the conditions in which man's productivity, health, mental and physical energy are at their highest efficiency. Both approaches may be combined, to show coinciding and complementary relationships, in defining desirable or disagreeable atmospheric and thermal conditions.

Effect of Weather on Human Body: Our daily life cycle comprises states of activity, fatigue and recovery. It is essential that the mind and body recover through recreation rest and sleep to counter balance. The mental and physical fatigue resulting from activities of the day. Unfavorable climatic conditions and the resulting stress on body often hinder this cycle and mind causes discomfort, loss of efficiency and may eventually lead to a breakdown of health. The effect of weather on living beings is therefore a factor of considerable importance. It is the task of the designer, architect or vastu expert to strive towards the optimum of total comfort. He has to consider both the physical as well as the emotional aspects of our environment.

Human thermal control is the dominant problem in tropical climates. Human response to the thermal environment does not only depend upon air temperature but also humidity, radiation and air movement. To understand the effect of these climatic factors, it is necessary to examine briefly the basic thermal processes of the human body i.e. heat gain and heat loss.

The body continuously produces heat. Most of the bio chemical processes involved in tissue building, energy conversion and muscular work are exothermic i.e. heat producing. All energy and material requirements of the body are supplied from the consumption and digestion of food. Of all the energy produced in the body, only about 20% are used while remaining 80% is 'surplus' heat and must be dissipated to the environment e.g. solar radiation or warm air that also has to be dissipated. The body can release heat to its environment by convection, radiation and evaporation and to some extent by conduction. Conduction depends on the temperature difference between the body surface and object the body is in direct contact with.

Elements of climate: A designer is generally interested in those aspects of climate, which affect human comfort in the use of the buildings. It includes averages, changes and extremes of temperature, the temperature differences between day and night, humidity, sky conditions, incoming and outgoing radiation, rainfall and its distribution, air movements – thunderstorms, dust storms, hurricanes. It is designer's job to analyze climatic information and present it in form that allows him to provide features, which are beneficial to the occupants of that building.

Vegetation: The elements of climate are incomplete without considering the character and abundance of plant life. Although generally regarded as a function of climate, vegetation influences the local or site climate. It is an important element in design of outdoor spaces, providing sun shading and protection from glare. For this we need a study and survey of native plants and trees – their shape and color, also their preferred orientation and situation. Factors governing the climate of a zone, which may cause local deviation, are:

1. Topography – i.e. slope, orientation, exposure, elevation, hills or valleys at or near the site.
2. Ground Surface – Whether natural or man – made, its reflectance, permeability and the soil temperature as these affect vegetation which in turn affects the climate (woods, shrubs, water, grass etc.)
3. Three dimensional objects: Such as trees, or tree belts, fences, walls and buildings as these may influence air movement, may cast a shadow and may subdivide the area into smaller units with different climatic features.

In general, the steps for the climatic planning comprises of:

1. Climate Data of a specific region should be analysed with the yearly characteristics of their constituent elements, such as temperature, relative humidity, radiation, and wind effects. The data, if necessary, should be adapted to the living level. And the modified effects of the micro-climate conditions should be considered.
2. Technological solutions may be sought, after the requirements are stated, to intercept the adverse and utilize the advantageous impacts at the right time and in adequate amount. This necessary function of a balanced shelter should be analysed by calculative methods :

   - In site selection most of the factors are variable. In general, sites, which show better characteristics in the winter – summer relationship, are more viable.

   - In orientation, the sun's heat is decisive both positively (in cold periods) and negatively (in hot periods). A balance can be found between the "under heated period", when we seek radiation, and the "overheated period", when we want to avoid it.

- Shading calculations are based on the maximum that throughout the year in under heated times, the sun should strike the building, and in overheated times, and the structure should be in shade. A chart of the sun's path, plus geometric and radiation calculations, can describe the effectiveness of shading devices.
- Housing forms and building shapes should conform to favourable or adverse impacts of the thermal environment; accordingly certain shapes are preferable to others in given surroundings.
- Air movements can be divided into the categorize of winds and breezes, according to their desirability. Winds occurring at under heated periods should be intercepted; cooling breezes should be utilized in overheated periods. Indoor air movement should satisfy bio-climatic needs.

3. Architectural application of the building of the findings of the first three steps must be developed and balanced according to the importance of the different elements. Climate balance begins at the site, and should be taken into consideration given to the individual dwelling units.

Building and Environment: The physical environment consists of many elements in a complex relationship. One can try to describe the environmental constituents as: light, sound, and climate, space, and animate. They all act directly upon the human body, which can either absorb them or try to counteract their effects. Physical and psychological reactions result from this struggle for biological equilibrium. Man strives for the point at which minimum expenditure of energy is needed to adjust himself to his environment. Conditions under which he succeeds in doing so can be defined as the "comfort zone", wherein most of his energy is freed for productivity.

The shelter is the main instrument for fulfilling the requirements of comfort. It modifies the natural environment to approach optimum conditions of liveability. It should filter, absorb, or repel environmental elements according to their beneficial or adverse contributions to man's comfort. Ideally, the satisfaction of all psychological needs would constitute the criterion of an environmentally balanced shelter. Here, however, only one element will be analysed – the feeling of thermal balance. Without it, any definition of comfort is impossible.

The major elements of climatic environment, which effect human comfort, can be categorized as: air temperature, radiation, air movement and humidity. There are others too, such as chemical differences, physical impurities electric content in the air. They act on man in a complex relationship, means by which the body exchanges heat with its surroundings can be classified into four main processes: radiation, conduction, convection and evaporation. It is estimated that radiation accounts for about 2/5 of the heat loss of the body, convection for 2/5 and evaporation 1/5; however, these proportions change with variations in the thermal conditions. The actual relative magnitude of body heat production and heat interchange with the environment may vary within wide limits. The vital processes of the body are accompanied by considerable energy exchange. This energy is derived from the oxidation of foodstuffs and is utilized with a gross efficiency of the order of 20%; the remaining 80% of the energy are expanded as heat. Even when the body is completely at rest and in warm surroundings its heat production does not fall below a certain minimum level – the basal metabolism.

The architect's problem is to produce an environment, which will not place undue stress upon the body's heat – compensation mechanism. The approach should be rephrased in terms of comfort; the presentation should be in graphic form; and, to be easily applicable, the data should derive from the empirical findings available to the practicing architect. Desirable air movements should be utilized for cooling in hot periods, and as a relief from vapour pressure during times of high absolute humidity. Conversely, air movement should be blocked and avoided by a bio-climatic analysis for the region, which divides the year into overheated and under heated during the cold season. The yardstick for evaluating wind movements is provided by a bio-climatic analysis for the region, which divides the year into overheated and under heated. Before investigating possible arrangements that will give wind protection or will utilize air movements beneficially, it is necessary to consider the orientation of the building.

All external heat impacts must pass through the building shell material; the process is comparable to the absorption of moisture by a porous material. Successive layers of the structure become 'saturated' with heat until finally the effect is felt on the inside surface. Anyone who has entered a large stone church on a hot summer day may have experienced it's comforting coolness. In such structures the large mass of the masonry materials absorbs and reflects the coolness of the previous night, resulting in a delayed temperature approximating a seasonal average. A similar effect is evident in such 'crypto-climatic' examples as the pyramids, where the interior space is negligible in relation to the immense mass of heavy material. The interior tomb chamber will constantly be close to the yearly average outdoor temperature. Historic houses sturdily built of heavy wall materials for reasons other than the thermal stability nevertheless react well from that standpoint. By comparison, the structures of today are extremely light and thin and the question of temperature balance arises urgently. Under many conditions light structures are quiet undesirable, being at the mercy of external forces just as light boats are tossed about on a high sea. The aim of this inquiry is to define the material requirements for an opaque shell, which, by damping and distribution, will balance the external thermal impacts of various regions and exposures. These qualities may be determined by investigating the processes and properties that allow for surface control, touching briefly the related problems of moisture and deterioration.

Ventilation: Ventilation consists an inlet of fresh air and maintaining a movement of air in the rooms and the building. For proper ventilation, windows should have minimum area of 1/8th of the floor area of the room and the aggregate area of the doors and windows should not be less than 1/4th of the floor area of the room. Windows should be provided 2'-6" above floor level. In addition to the doors and windows, ventilators should be provided having a total area of 4% of floor area. Ventilation serve as good exit for inside air and should be provided as near to the ceiling as possible within 60cm (2 feet) from the ceiling. The area of each ventilator should not be less than .3 sq. m (3 sq. ft.)

In living room, at least two windows should be provided one in each of the opposite walls, if that is not possible, there should be a at least two window one in each of the adjoining walls. Bath rooms, toilets, kitchens should have at least one window of adequate size.

Sick Building Syndrome and Extreme Climatic Conditions

If the building is not designed considering climatic parameters, it can certainly lead to Sick Building Syndrome. For example a house in Leh-Ladakh may require some extreme considerations otherwise survival in such a place would be difficult for extreme cold months. Such a building would not have comfortable environment and would lead to unhealthy internal bio-climate. Similarly if a building is not designed in Jaisalmer considering the extreme heat, it can again lead to unhealthy internal bio-climate and uncomfortable environment for the residents. It is very important for buildings to adapt to the climatic conditions and create an internal healthy and comfortable bio-climate. The solution to extreme climatic conditions in a building is through wise, sensitive and careful creation of building as discussed earlier in the chapter.

Electro Magnetic Radiations and Sick Building Syndrome

The Sun's Electromagnetic Waves

Electromagnetic Waves are waves of electric and magnetic force. They are generated by the Oscillation of electric charges. The strength of the Electromagnetic wave varies in space and time with alternating crests and troughs. The Sun's Electromagnetic spectrum consists of bands of different wavelengths. The chief kinds of electromagnetic waves are in order of increasing wavelength- gamma rays, X – rays, Ultra violet light, visible light, infra red rays, microwaves & radio waves. The direction of magnetic force in all electromagnetic waves is perpendicular to the direction in which the wave is moving. The direction of electric force is perpendicular to both the direction of magnetic force and the direction of wave motion. The strength of magnetic force always equals the strength of electric force.

Electric fields are created by differences in voltage: the higher the voltage, the stronger will be the resultant field. **Magnetic fields** are created when electric current flows: the greater the current, the stronger the magnetic field. An electric field will exist even when there is no current flowing. If current does flow, the strength of the magnetic field will vary with power consumption but the electric field strength will be constant.

Electromagnetic fields are present everywhere in our environment but are invisible to the human eye. Electric fields are produced by the local build-up of electric charges in the atmosphere associated with thunderstorms. The earth's magnetic field causes a compass needle to orient in a North-South direction and is used by birds and fish for navigation.

Electromagnetic radiation has been around since the birth of the universe; light is its most familiar form. Electric and magnetic fields are part of the spectrum of electromagnetic radiation which extends from static electric and magnetic fields, through radio frequency and infrared radiation, to X-rays.

Uses of electromagnetic waves:

- Gamma rays and are used for treatment of cancer.
- X – rays are used for treatment of cancer and diagnose internal disorders.
- Ultra Violet rays are used in Sun lamps and fluorescent light and as a disinfectant.
- Infra red rays, which are given off by hot objects, are used in infrared lamps to treat skin disease.
- Micro waves are used to cook food.
- Radio waves are used in radio and T.V. broadcasting.

How to deduct/identify the excess radiation?

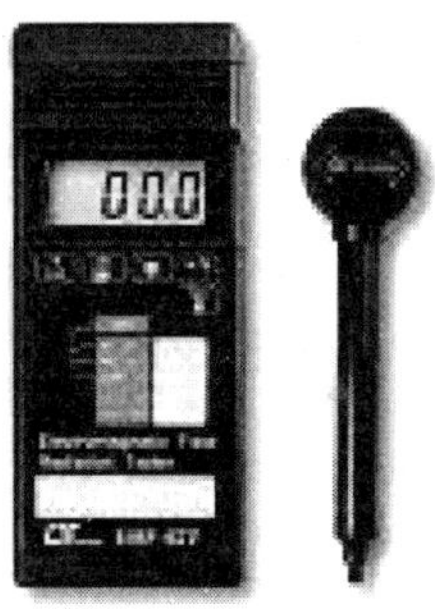

EM Radiation Tester

At present Europe is more aware on aspects of health related to radiations in comparison to America. In India, there is very little awareness about harm from radiations. Scientists have developed precise scientific instrumentation to actually quantify subtle magnetic field fluctuations in bedrooms, and even in the U.S... Medical researchers are accepting the role of very weak magnetic fields in physical health.

Presently EMF radiation tester is used to detect electromagnetic radiations in a confined or open space.

There are generic guidelines by US EPA on wise use of gadgets. The danger zone is subject to the product and electric consumption.

Danger Zones EMF Levels from Common Sources in Milligauss (mG) Recommended Safety Levels 0.5mG-2.5mG		
SOURCE	up to 4 inches	at 3 feet
Blender	50-220	0.3-3
Clothes Washer	8-200	0.1-4
Coffee Maker	6-29	0.1
Computer	4-20	2-5
Flourescent Lamp	400-4,000	0.1-5
Hair Dryer	60-20,000	0.1-6
Microwave Oven	100-500	1-25
Television	5-100	0.1-6
Vacuum Cleaner	230-1,300	3-40
Airplane	50 mG	
Source: USA Environmental Protection Agency		

Electromagnetic Fields and Public Health

Base Stations and Wireless Technologies

Mobile phones- a wireless technology relies upon an extensive network of fixed antennas, or base stations, relaying information with radio-frequency (RF) signals. Over 1.4 million base stations exist worldwide and the number is increasing significantly with the introduction of third generation technology.

Other wireless networks that allow high-speed internet access and services, such as wireless local area networks (WLANs), are also increasingly common in homes, offices, and many public places. As the number of base stations and local wireless networks increases, so does the RF exposure of the population. There has been concern about possible health consequences from exposure to the RF fields produced by wireless technologies. This fact sheet reviews the scientific evidence on the health effects from continuous low-level human exposure to base stations and other local wireless networks.

Media or anecdotal reports of cancer clusters around mobile phone base stations have heightened public concern. It should be noted that geographically, cancers are unevenly distributed among any population. Given the widespread presence of base stations in the environment, it is expected that possible cancer clusters will occur near base stations merely by chance. Moreover, the reported cancers in these clusters are often a collection of different types of cancer with no common characteristics and hence unlikely to have a common cause.

Scientific evidence on the distribution of cancer in the population can be obtained through carefully planned and executed epidemiological studies. Over the past 15 years, studies examining a potential relationship between RF transmitters and cancer have been published. These studies have not provided evidence that RF exposure from the transmitters increases the risk of cancer. Likewise, long-term animal studies have not established an increased risk of cancer from exposure to RF fields, even at levels that are much higher than produced by base stations and wireless networks.

One of the main characteristics which define an electromagnetic field (EMF) is its frequency or its corresponding wavelength. Fields of different frequencies interact with the body in different ways. One can imagine electromagnetic waves as series of very regular waves that travel at an enormous speed, the speed of light.

Electromagnetic Fields at Low Frequencies

Electric fields exist whenever a positive or negative electrical charge is present. They exert forces on other charges within the field. The strength of the electric field is measured in volts per meter (V/m). Any electrical wire that is charged will produce an associated electric field. This field exists even when there is no current flowing. The higher the voltage, the stronger the electric field at a given distance from the wire.

Electric fields are strongest close to a charge or charged conductor, and their strength rapidly diminishes with distance from it. Conductors such as metal shield them very effectively. Other materials, such as building materials and trees, provide some shielding capability. Therefore, the electric fields from power lines outside the house are reduced by walls, buildings, and trees. When power lines are buried in the ground, the electric fields at the surface are hardly detectable.

Magnetic fields arise from the motion of electric charges. The strength of the magnetic field is measured in amperes per meter (A/m); more commonly in electromagnetic field research, scientists specify a related quantity, the flux density instead. In contrast to electric fields, a magnetic field is only produced once a device is switched on and current flows. The higher the current, the greater is the strength of the magnetic field.

Like electric fields, magnetic fields are strongest close to their origin and rapidly decrease at greater distances from the source. Magnetic fields are not blocked by common materials such as the walls of buildings. Mobile telephones, television and radio transmitters and radar produce RF fields. These fields are used to transmit information over long distances and form the basis of telecommunications as well as radio and television broadcasting all over the world. Microwaves are RF fields at high frequencies in the GHz range.

WHO, through the International EMF Project, has established a program to monitor the EMF scientific literature, to evaluate the health effects from exposure to EMF in the range from 0 to 300 GHz, to provide advice about possible EMF hazards and to identify suitable mitigation measures? It is recognized that some of the more extreme frequencies are harmful (x-rays and ultraviolet rays), but what about the constant bombardment from domestic and office appliances? Overhead and underground high voltage cables, mobile phones etc. The most consistent effect of electromagnetic stress is on the human body both mental & physical.

Effects and Resonances on Human Beings

Our body has its own electrical and magnetic system. Electrical energy created in the brain regulates complex biological process. Our bodies electrics can be distributed and disrupted by environmental electromagnetic fields, natural (geo-pathos stress) and man-made (electro stress). Radiations from nature can be through sun or earth.

Geopathic stress are radiations affecting immune function. Any natural weaknesses or genetic disorders are amplified. Most significant consistent effect of electro stress on the human system is on the body's ability to absorb nutrients. Every client whose body is detrimentally affected by electro magnetic disturbances has a compressed nutrient absorption rate. Once the source of electro magnetic disturbances is deactivated or removed, nutrient absorption rate rapidly returns to optimal levels.

Electro magnetic field are invisible to the naked eye, but it shows harmful effect on our body, so electromagnetic field have been part of the earth's environment. Resonances occurs between the earth's molten iron nickel core and the charged gases of the ionosphere. They pulse at definite frequencies (between 0.1 and 25 HZ mostly at about 10 Hz) and act as regulators for the biological time clocks of all living creatures. If a man or any living animal or plant is shielded from these fields for any length of time the result is discomfort and ill health.

Anything which uses electricity for its operation generates a field, whether it is AC or DC. Automotive currents are in general more harmful because they pulse Due to geo and environment stress there can be impact on our life. Our body has an energy axis which is aligned with the centre of the body, when it is resonates with the flow of energies in the space. When disturbed, the axis moves out and causes loss of immunity and health disorders over a period of time. Almost all radiations, known to mankind have a wavelength of less than 20 cm. Scientific reports have suggested that exposure to electromagnetic fields emitted from these devices could have adverse health effects, such as cancer, reduced fertility, memory loss, and adverse changes in the behaviour and development of children.

Health Effects of Electro Magnetic Radiations

The following list represents diseases and health problems that are either a direct result of electromagnetic radiation poisoning or are closely associated with it. Keep in mind that all health issues will be affected to some degree by exposure to EMF radiation, whether electric, magnetic, wireless or ionizing radiation, since it weakens the immune system, stresses the body and damages healthy cells.

- Cancer
- Alzheimer's
- Parkinson's
- Fibromyalgia
- Chronic Fatigue
- Daily Headaches
- Brain Cancer
- Lyme Disease
- Asthma
- Heart Problems
- Chest Pain
- Insomnia
- Allergies
- Electrosensitivity (ES)/Electromagnetic Hypersensitivitiy (EHS)
- Multiple Sclerosis
- High Blood Pressure
- Digestive Disorders
- Migraine Headaches
- Brain Tumors
- Leukemia – General
- Lymphoblastic Leukemia
- Birth Defects
- Miscarriages
- Stress
- Nausea
- Rheumatoid Arthritis
- Lupus
- Fatigue
- Skin Conditions – Burning, Rashes, Pain
- Tinnitus and Other Audible Noises
- Chronic Pain
- Erratic Pulse, and
- Weak Immune System etc.

Factors that Encourage the Dangers of Electromagnetic Radiation

Though every person's cells are affected by electromagnetic radiation, each is affected at different 'speeds'. Here are some of the factors that encourage a faster or stronger reaction to EMF exposures.

- High stress levels
- Low iodine levels
- Heavy metal toxicity
- High total EMF exposure
- Having other pre-existing health problems
- Weakened immune system

Remedy and Safety Precaution

Now days electromagnetic radiations are almost unavoidable. The magnetic fields easily, penetrate brick wall, R.C.C. slab, stonewall or roof & human bodies and as of now, no protective shield is available with such a pervasive yet mysterious force around us, there's not much we can do to totally eliminate EMFs exposure. Although there are claims of innumerable companies who create EMF shielding paints and sheets. There are simple ways of minimizing our potential risks. Below mentioned are some of the suggestions:

a) There should be an approximate distance of 4-6 feet between television and bed.

b) Switch off your mobile at night and reduce the radiations in the bedroom, or else keep the on silent mode outside your bedroom.

c) Don't allow children to peer through the doors of microwave ovens when they are on.

d) Pregnant women should avoid using video- display terminals (VDTs).

e) Avoid living in areas where EMF exposure could be high.

f) People at greatest risk are utility workers & those near transmission lines

g) Use M.S. conduct pipe 16 gage for building wiring & earth both end properly.

h) All your electric, electronic items must be properly earthed.

i) Switch off you bedroom wiring from the main in the night before going to sleep.

j) After use immediately switch off from main all your electric and electronic gadgets.

Geopathic Radiations and Sick Building Syndrome

This chapter has been prepared in reference to thesis of our Ph.D student Dr. Sonal Kiran Lavingia submitted to Zoroastrian College as "GEOPATHIC STRESS & TREATMENT AS PER VASTU PRINCIPLES" in year 2009 and "CANCER AND PSYCHOSOMATIC DISORDER DUE TO GEOPATHIC STRESS" in year 2011.

The word Geobiology comes from the two words Geo -- meaning (Earth) and Bio – meaning (Life). Geobiology is the study of the earth structure, and the influence it has on all life forms existing on the planet. Geobiology basically understands the impact of different forms of geo-energies on various aspects of life (physical, mental, emotional, intellectual and spiritual) above it. In simple words it is a clear relationship between *terrestrial space* (land or earth) and *inner space* (living being). **Geobiology is a study of gases, vibrations, energies or radiations emitting from land and their impact on living organisms or life above it.** The job of the agrobiologists is to detect harmful elements of land and its related energies, to rebalance the living space and to raise the level of positive vibrations, in order to allow the body to recharge itself. It has been scientifically demonstrated that a long stay in a disturbed location, has a definite effect on the electromagnetic functioning of our cells, devitalizes our organism and weakens our immunity system.

In ancient times, architecture was not only a creation of form to define a particular space, but was inherently a sacred form to take care of the subtle effects of the environment, both natural and built up on the human body. So our ancestors created forms that were in harmony with the creation that surround us, forms that live not in time but that have out grown time and live in eternity.

Today Geobiology dedicates itself to an investigation of the principles on which certain laws are based. The earth consists of several layers, the core, the mantle and the crust and is surrounded by the atmosphere. It is very important to study which material the earth is consisted of and the energies that are present in the same. Geologists have looked at the earth, divided by major rock types, by links to engineering, chemistry, physics and biology, by a focus on specific environment or resources, or by a focus on the static and dynamic properties of earth materials i.e. mineralogy, geomorphology and structural geology.

The influences generated by the earth are generally brought about by the earth's magnetic field and local geological characteristics. Earth has positive and negative poles and is surrounded by its own magnetic field (geomagnetic field) at the rate 7.8 beats / second. The intensity of this field varies according to the location and the hour of the day.

The human being is like an antenna between the earth and the sky. The human body is submitted to a continuous exchange of energy between these two poles and the earth sky flow nourishes it energetically, for its survival. In nature this flow of energy is called cosmos telluric channel while this flow of energies in humans is referred to as global balance. Being a very hypersensitive and highly sophisticated antenna, the human body receives and transmits endless information all the time, though most of the time not being aware about it. This unconscious information is received through resonance and stocked in our cells, and influences the functioning of our bodies. When two bodies have similar wave lengths and frequencies, they have an instant communication through resonance no matter what the distance between the two of them is.

Earth is a living being with elements, similar to our body. It has 70% of water; it has meridians, veins, articulations and subtle bodies. That is why our body communicates so well with the Earth through resonance. The earth is threaded with energy lines or meridians of electromagnetic energy that have a powerful influence on living beings. Scientists have proven this invisible energy passes through all matter, affecting every living system on the planet, in either a negative or positive way. Man is an electromagnetic creature with every cell in the living system an electrical battery. The electrical system is reflected even more subtly as the human aura that is a photographable and measurable electrical field.

It has been noticed that lands unsuitable for human habitation creates physical and physiological illnesses for residents at different levels. Buildings constructed on degraded or barren lands without treatment can lead to Sick Building Syndrome.

The Structure of Geobiology

The purpose of Geobiology is to provide the data to enable us create a habitat as near to natural living conditions as possible, taking into account the need for comfort provided by old and new technologies favourable to the environment. As per Geobiology there are two kinds of underground water veins, primary water and aquifer water flowing in earth. The first one is water that comes up from the deepest parts of the earth for the first time, It is known as healing water and is the water that flows out of earth in well known hot thermal stations as for example in Yellowstone.

The second kind of underground water veins is aquifer water. The natural radioactivity above these veins is higher than usual, and the magnetic field is very low. Its influence affects a height of 100 meters. The friction of the underground water on the rocks creates a very strong vibration on the surface. This vibration becomes more noxious if the water is polluted. Its presence can be noticed above surface on the vegetation; trees grow diagonally trying to avoid the vibration, wholes in planted hedges. Lightning often touch earth where two underground water veins cross each other.

Geopathic emissions also relate to physical properties of soil. The physical level deals with all the known effects related to the quality of the ground (ie geological fault, water streams, Radon...etc.). Soil science looks at the outer skin of terrestrial earth.

Soil

Soil plays an essential role in supporting life on earth and is a scarce resource of great economic value. It responds quickly to environmental changes and indeed bears the human impact on the land surface. Soil is one of the three major natural resources, alongside air and water. It is one of the marvellous products of nature and without which there would be no life.

Soil is a natural body consisting of layers (Soil horizons) of mineral constituents of variable thickness which differ from the parent material in their morphological, physical, chemical and mineralogical characteristics. It is composed and altered by chemical and environmental processes that include weathering and erosion and is a mixture of organic constituents that are solid gaseous and gaseous states.

Soil Selection

Soil formation greatly depends on the climatic conditions, and soils from different climate zones, show distinctive characteristics. Soil is populated by an amazing variety of living creatures, ranging from tiny microbes such

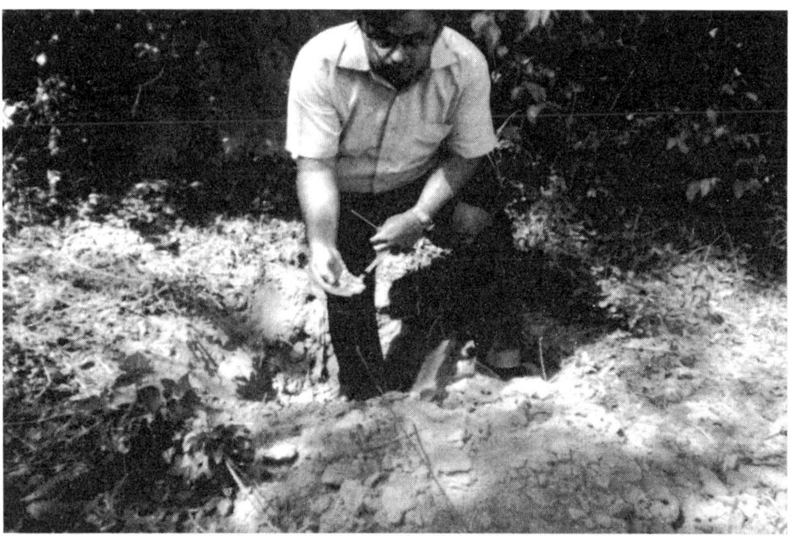

as bacteria and fungi (microbeasts), to smaller insects such as centipedes and other animals such as worms (minibeasts) and larger animals such as moles and rabbits. Bacteria, an essential group of soil micro-organisms, are responsible for much of the decomposition of organic material in soils. They are usually present in top soils in very large numbers and play an important role in converting more inert forms of nitrogen to ones that can more readily be taken up by plants.

Soil is a mixture of mineral and organic materials plus air and water. The contents of soil vary from location to location, and are constantly changing. There are many different kinds and types of soils. Each kind has certain characteristics and has specific colours and compositions. Different kinds of soils support different types of plant growths, and also determine how well that plant life grow. Soil is formed slowly, but can be destroyed very easily.

Types of Soils

The first impression when viewing a particular soil is its colour, and can be classified by the composition of clay, silt, and sand within it. The study of Geobiology says that a particular place can either make us prone to disease or depression or can even lift us to more subtle levels of vibrations, strengthening our body and spirit, depending on its characteristics. Soil is a living system and a variety of soil organisms live in it. These include bacteria, fungi, micro arthropods, nematodes, earthworms and insects. These organisms live on soil organic matter or other soil organisms and perform a number of vital processes in the soil. Other organisms are involved in transformation of inorganic molecules. Very few soil organisms are pests.

Soil chemistry is concerned with the availability of elements for plant uptake as well as the presence in soil of elements and chemical compounds that might be present at levels that are detrimental to plants and soil organisms. Some elements in the soil are nutrients and are essential for plant growth. Other elements are not essential and may be toxic to plants. The availability of elements for plant uptake is affected by soil pH and reactions of the elements with soil particles and organic matter.

Physical properties like Structure and Texture of the soil, and processes such as Erosion of the soil, can affect the soil fertility. Structure is the amount of aggregation and pores in soil and texture is the proportion of clay and sand particles in soil. Both of these affect soil fertility by affecting water movement through the soil, root penetration and water logging. Erosion is an important physical process that decreases soil fertility. When soil structure and texture are unfavourable for water movement through soil water erosion and water logging may be increased. Soil salinity is a chemical property but can affect soil physical fertility by decreasing the movement of water through the soil.

Soil pollution is defined as the build-up in soils of persistent toxic compounds, chemicals, salts, radioactive materials, or disease causing agents, which have adverse effects on plant growth and animal health.

The effects of soil pollution are:

- Insufficient Oxygen in the soil,
- Acidic soils may burn the plants,
- Bugs may go and start an infestation in the soil,
- Plant-growth is affected,
- Not enough drainage,
- New soil diseases develop every year, and
- Not enough moisture in the soil.

Soil pollution results from the build up of:

- Contaminants,
- Toxic Compounds,
- Radioactive Materials,
- Salts,
- Chemicals, and
- Cancer-causing agents.

The most common soil pollutants are

- Hydrocarbons,
- Heavy metals (Cadmium, Lead, Chromium, Copper, Zinc, Mercury and Arsenic),
- Herbicides,
- Pesticides,
- Oils, and
- Tars, etc.

Land Degradation

Degraded land demands attention or due treatment before use. A user should be very careful while selecting a land. There are various reasons of land degradation. Approximately, 28 per cent of it belongs to the category of forest degraded area, 56 per cent of it is water eroded area and the rest is affected by saline and alkaline deposits. Some human activities such as deforestation, over grazing, mining and quarrying too have contributed significantly in land degradation.

- Mining sites are abandoned after excavation work is complete leaving deep scars and traces of over-burdening. In states like Jharkhand, Chhattisgarh, Madhya Pradesh and Orissa deforestation due to mining have caused severe land degradation.
- In states like Gujarat, Rajasthan, Madhya Pradesh and Maharashtra overgrazing is one of the main reasons for land degradation.
- In the states of Punjab, Haryana, western Uttar Pradesh, over

irrigation is responsible for land degradation due to water logging leading to increase in salinity and alkalinity in the soil.

- ❖ The mineral processing like grinding of limestone for cement industry and calcite and soapstone for ceramic industry generate huge quantity of dust in the atmosphere.
- ❖ It retards the process of infiltration of water into the soil after it settles down on the land.
- ❖ In recent years, industrial effluents as waste have become a major source of land and water pollution in many parts of the country.

Classification of Soils

On the basis of the factors responsible for soil formation, colour, thickness, texture, age and properties, the soils of India can be classified in different types.

- ❖ Alluvial Soil
- ❖ Black Soil
- ❖ Red and Yellow Soil
- ❖ Laterite Soil
- ❖ Arid Soil
- ❖ Forest Soil

Importance Fertile of Land

Ideally a fertile land without Geobiologiocal faults should be chosen for a construction site. Fertile land has fertile soil in it. Fertile soil has the following properties:

- It is rich in nutrients necessary for basic plant nutrition, including nitrogen,
- It contains sufficient minerals (trace elements) for plant nutrition, including boron, chlorine, cobalt, copper, iron, manganese, magnesium, molybdenum, sulphur, and zinc.
- It contains soil organic matter that improves soil structure and soil moisture retention.
- Soil pH is in the range 6.0 to 6.8 for most plants but some prefer acid or alkaline conditions.
- Good soil structure, creating well drained soil, but some soils are wetter (as for producing rice) or drier (as for producing plants susceptible to fungi or rot, such as agave).
- A range of micro-organisms that support plant growth.
- It often contains large amounts of topsoil.

In lands used for agriculture and other human activities, fertile soil typically arises from the use of soil conservation practices. Basically, soil fertility refers to the ability of a soil to supply plant nutrients.

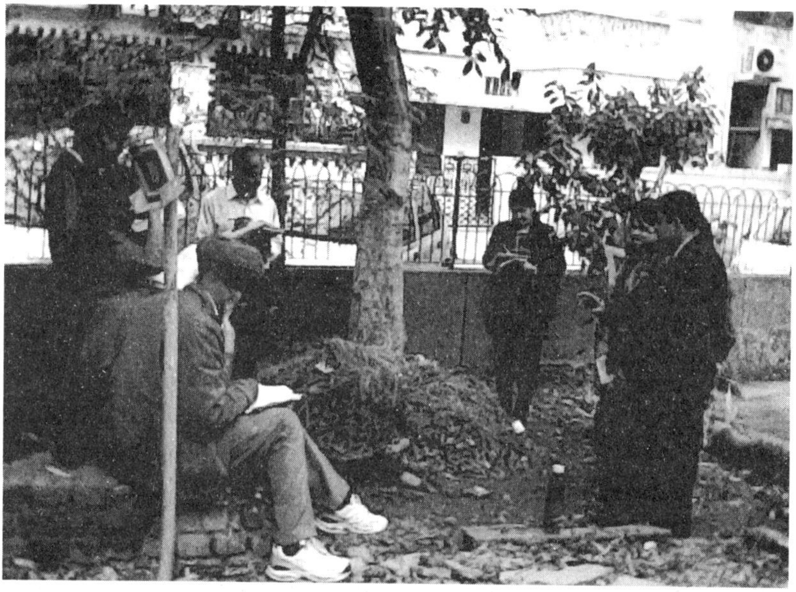

Checking Fertility of Soil

Soil Testing

Soil may be defined as a thin layer of earth's crust which serves as a natural medium for growth of plants. It is the unconsolidated mineral matter that has been subjected to, and influenced by, genetic and environmental factors such as parent material, climate, organisms and topography all acting over a period of time. Soil differs from the parent material in the morphological, physical, chemical and biological properties. Some soils are red, some are black; some are deep and some are shallow; some are coarse textured and some are fine-textured. They serve as a reservoir of nutrients and water for crops, provide mechanical anchorage and favourable tilt. The components of soil are mineral matter, organic matter, water and air, the proportions of which vary and together form a system for plant growth. Soil is defined as the top layer of the earth's crust. It is formed by mineral particles, organic matter, water, air and living organisms. It is in fact an extremely complex, variable and living medium. The interface between the earth, the air and the water, soil is a non-renewable resource which performs many vital functions: food and other biomass production, storage, filtration and transformation of many substances including water, carbon, and nitrogen. Soil has a role as a habitat and gene pool, serves as a platform for human activities, landscape and heritage and acts as a provider of raw materials. These functions are worthy of protection because of their socio-economic as well as environmental importance.

A soil test provides information about pH, lime requirements and variable phosphorous, Potassium, Calcium, magnesium etc. There are different types of tests as per the project's requirement. Soil is alive and constantly changing. After studying the soil testing reports, balancing materials can be applied to neutralize the soil as per the requirements. We can use soil testing to find out the different geopathically stressed sections or zones and trying to know the exact composition of the soil obtained from that sections. Study of such zones may help us to rectify the soil and thus it may be beneficial to the society.

We know that under the Earth, we may find soil to be acidic in some areas, whereas dry or even watery in some areas. This does have impact on the chemical changes that may take place on adding certain minerals to the soil, which can be evaluated by the soil testing and hence can guide us to use the appropriate minerals in the soil of the faulty zones in order to rectify the faults.

Various reports show the electro conductivity in some samples too high. TDS composition is also high in geopathically stressed lands. The HCO3, CL, NO3, S04 shows remarkable difference in their readings. Soil electrical conductivity, which is known as EC, is the ability of soil to conduct electrical current. EC is expressed in MilliSiemens per meter (mS/m). Traditionally, soil scientists used EC to measure soil salinity. The conduction of electricity in soil takes place through the moisture-filled pores that occur between individual soils particles. EC readings correlate strongly to soil grain size or texture. Sand has low conductivity, silts have a medium conductivity and clays have a high conductivity. The art of using electrical conductivity knows what physical or chemical soil property causes changes in soil EC.

If the quantum of salts and minerals in underground water is more than the prescribed limits, that water is polluted. For instance, additional quantity of fluoride can pollute groundwater. The presence of salts and minerals should be within the prescribed limits. Groundwater can become polluted, or contaminated. It can become polluted from leaky underground tanks that store gasoline, leaky landfills, or when people apply too much fertilizer or pesticides on their fields or lawns.

Pesticides and fertilizers used in agriculture and weed killers from road verges are washed off when it rains. They may go into ground-water used for public water supplies, polluting them. They may go into lakes and rivers and harm living organisms there. Natural contaminants can come from many conditions in the watershed or in the ground. Water moving through rocks and soils may pick up magnesium, calcium, and chlorides.

Some ground water contains dissolved elements such as arsenic, boron, selenium, or radon—a gas formed by the natural breakdown of radioactive uranium in soil. Whether these natural contaminants are health problems depends on the amount of substance present.

Some naturally occurring sources of pollution include:

Micro-organisms. Bacteria, viruses, parasites, and other micro-organisms are sometimes found in water. Shallow wells—those with water close to ground level—are at most risk. Runoff, or water flowing over the land surface, may pick up these pollutants from wildlife and soils. This is often the case after flooding.

Salinity is a highly important problem in arid and semi-arid regions. Consequently, the analysis of soil salinity plays a crucial role in environmental sciences. Electrical conductivity (EC) is a measurement of the dissolved material in an aqueous solution, which relates to the ability of the material to conduct electrical current through it. EC is measured in units called Siemens per unit area (e.g. mS/cm, or MilliSiemens per centimetre), and the higher the dissolved material in a water or soil sample, the higher the EC will be in that material. Temperate streams and lakes, especially those with a significant groundwater contribution, generally have higher electrical conductivities. EC measurements can vary greatly and are affected by several environmental factors including, climate, local biota (plants and animals), bedrock and surgical geology, as well as human impacts on the land. High conductivity may indicates high concentrations of ions/nutrients, therefore high soil salt content.

Geopathic Stress

'Geopathic' literally means 'earth-associated illness. The earth's magnetic field is constantly fluctuating and this causes natural radiation to rise through the ground. Natural causes of geopathic stress are nowadays compounded by the electromagnetic fields generated by mobile phones, microwaves, cars and so on, which produce stress. Geopathic Stress is caused by the detrimental effects of negative earth energies which pass through walls, windows, and closed doors. These energies are not stable and can change with the seasons or even with the time of the day and can be distorted by building works carried out even at some distance away.

Geopathic stress is a form of trauma caused by disturbed or anomalous energies within the earth's mantle or within the soil. The earth is surrounded by an energy grid which contains and transmits vital forces. This grid is essential for life and is a part of the background radiation which supports life. Within the earth there is naturally occurring beneficial radiation but when the earth is disturbed, e.g. by digging, including building and construction work or due to any natural disasters such as earth quakes, landslide, this balance can be altered and the harmful energies can be released underneath the ground surface. Geopathic stress therefore represents a distortion of the natural frequency which can sometimes be observed visibly in nature- Eggplants failing to thrive, trees taking on peculiar angles and trunk developments. In contrast some special plants seem to positively flourish in areas where geopathic stress has been detected.

Medical professionals seem to all agree that CHRONIC STRESS is one of the biggest killers in the world. Chronic stress means the body is out of balance and the immune system is weak which allows the body to become a breeding ground for any sickness, anxiety, depression, gastrointestinal disorders, etc. Today the World Health Organization considers that 30% of all buildings are 'sick' buildings.

Van Allen Radiation Belt

The Van Allen Radiation Belt is a torus of energetic charged particles (plasma) around Earth, held in place by Earth's magnetic field. Apollo astronauts who travelled to the moon spent very little time in the belts but probably have a slightly higher risk of cancer during their trip. NASA said that they deliberately timed Apollo launches, and used lunar transfer orbits that only skirted the edge of the belt over the equator to minimize the radiation. Besides, there have been nuclear tests in space that have caused artificial radiation belts. Starfish Prime, a high altitude nuclear test created an artificial radiation belt that damaged or destroyed as many as one third of the satellites in low earth orbit at the time.

Geopathic Stress and Scientific Researches

In 1929, Baron Gustav Fresher von Pohl discovered that many cases of human illness and disease in animals, plants and trees were related to underground fissures and streams of water emitted energy vertically to the surface. He suspected that the velocity of the water was the most important factor in the strength of this disease-inducing energy. Further, he discovered that unusually high levels of natural electric currents occurred where underground water fissures crossed at different levels.

Ionization under the Beds of Cancer Patients

In 1939, Pierre Cody of Le Havre used an electrometer to measure ionization under the beds of cancer victims and discovered very high readings vertically above the surface of the ground. Another researcher in more recent times, Kate Basher, an Austrian teacher, has worked extensively with geopathically disturbed zones, and has listed 11,000 cases of illness which she believes were initiated in these areas. She helped the sufferers to move their beds or working positions to a more suitable area, with extremely beneficial results. Her research has centred partly on the unpleasant influences of what she called 'malign earth energies' were having on children at school, not only with respect to their health, but also to their ability to learn. She found that 95% of children who were unsuccessful in school, who were slow learners, or lethargic, were difficult to handle, or hyperactive, had been found in the areas of geopathic stress. Kate believes that children in a class ought to change the position of their desks, perhaps every three to four weeks; one row of children alternating with the adjacent row, so that no child should suffer what may be a stressful environment for any long period.

A recent survey by Christopher McNamee of the People's Research Centre, Alston, has revealed that gypsies and travelling people have a surprisingly low level of illness. When asked about incidences of cancer in their relatives, he found that it is less than 1%, against 25-33% mortality in the rest of the population. Heart disease and other serious illnesses so prevalent in our society are also very low in them. Their general lifestyle can hardly be attributed to their well-being, as they smoke, drink alcohol and ignore health foods and special diets. He also believes that illness is primarily a disease of location, and that the travelling people's nomadic lifestyle means that they are unlikely to stay long in a highly stressed area, and if they do happen to camp in one, they are intuitive enough to leave the area after a very short time.

Professor Herbert Koenig of Munich found that a person's blood sedimentation rate changes when he sleeps or stays in a geopathically stressed zone. He felt that this could lead eventually to heart disorders, if nothing was done. Further studies in German and American cities by Egon Eckert of Newton showed that most cases were distributed along high power lines. The conjunction of high power lines, underground water streams and Hartmann grid crossing should be considered as extreme perturbation of the ambient field. It should be essential to have a correct positioning of beds in places where people have a diminished resistance and health such as hospitals.

According to B Merz (Institute of Geobiology of Chardonnay, Lausanne in Switzerland) just as a place can make us prone to disease or depression, another can lift us to more subtle levels of vibration, strengthening our body and spirit. Such places were sought after throughout history and held as sacred. Some are natural wonders like Ayers Rock; the Aborigines have long known this, the Grand Canyon, the Matterhorn and countless other places on this planet which inspire the millions of modern pilgrims. In India the holy places like rishikesh, haridwar, badrinath, amaranth, dwarkadhish and many more have been supported by positive land vibrations.

Researchers and scientists have noted that Geopathic Stress does not necessarily cause illness but seems to lower a person's immune system, so if they are sleeping in an area that is geopathically stressed, their body is not getting a proper chance to repair. In recent years the rapid proliferation of artificial sources of radio electric frequencies has become a cause for concern. It has surpassed many times the production of natural sources.

It is interesting that where Geopathic stress has been found, the occupants of that property have often noted that since moving there, their health has deteriorated, their sleep has not been restful and previously happy families are encountering more arguments or a sense of unhappiness. It has also been found that houses where geopathic stress is found are often harder to sell and return to the market regularly as people have not been comfortable there. Positive relationships with neighbours may have also suffered. Geopathic stress in the work place also seems to generate its own tensions with a work force who can be argumentative and uncooperative, or who may not stay in the job long or there is a higher incidence of sick leave.

Geopathic Stress and Animals

Some of the researches reveal that some animals like cats seem to be drawn to Geopathic stress whereas many birds tend to be repelled by it. Cats are very sensitive and prefer the spots to sit and sleep which are stressed while on the contrary if a Dog, cow or a horse continuously refuses to stay or sleep at a place, indicates negative radiations from land and calls for further geo biological diagnosis.

Reasons of Geopathic Stress:

1. Certain mineral deposits
2. Underground Cavities
3. Underground debris of dead
4. Movements of the continental tectonic plates
5. Changes at the core level of earth
6. Land-burn due to massive fire or other natural calamities
7. Establishment of heavy machinery for years
8. Buildings constructed on clutter
9. Buried utility pipes, soak pit or septic tank
10. Man-made disturbance
11. Mines-rail cuttings
12. Criss-cross water veins
13. Black streams/Black spots etc.

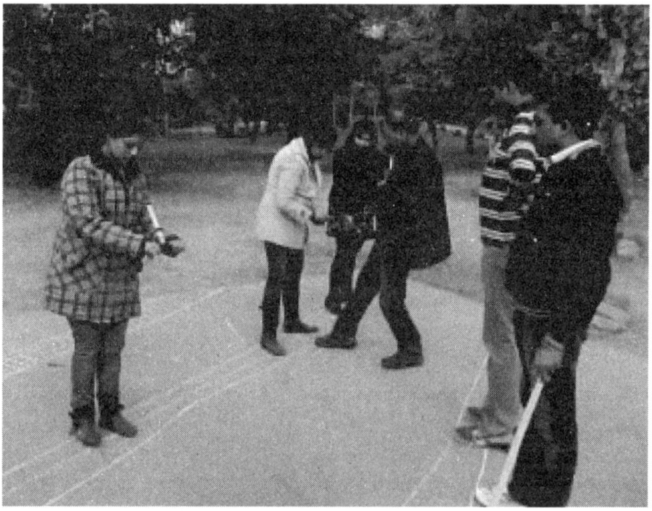

Finding Grids

The Hartmann Grid and Curry Grid

Hartmann grids were discovered in 1950 by a German medical doctor; Ernst Hartmann. The lines form a grid around the earth running North to South and East to West and extended to a height of 60-600 feet –The North-South lines appear approximately every 2m and the East West lines appear every 2.5m. In reality the distance between the lines varies from place to place. In Delhi the distance between the lines is generally around 1.5m. According to Dr. Hartmann the worst place that a person can sleep or work is over a Hartmann knot, where two Hartmann lines cross. These disported fields of radiation are harmful to living organisms and produce Geopathic stress. These dynamic environments are sensitive to the rhythms of the hours and seasons.

The crossing points or nodes of these lines are considered to be unhealthy if one is to remain over them for long periods of time as in a bed or at a work station. The regularity of the Hartmann grid can also be affected by man-made disturbances such as high tension power lines, roads etc.

The effect of a crossing or knot in the Hartmann grid can be amplified by other local characteristics such as geological fault making that particular spot potentially dangerous. According to Prof. Endros trees growing on the crossing of the grid are prone to being hit by lightning, especially if they are near or over an underground stream. Most trees or plants showing deformities are found on such "knots" of the Hartmann grid.

Further studies in German and American cities by Egon Eckert of Newton showed that most cases were distributed along high power lines. The

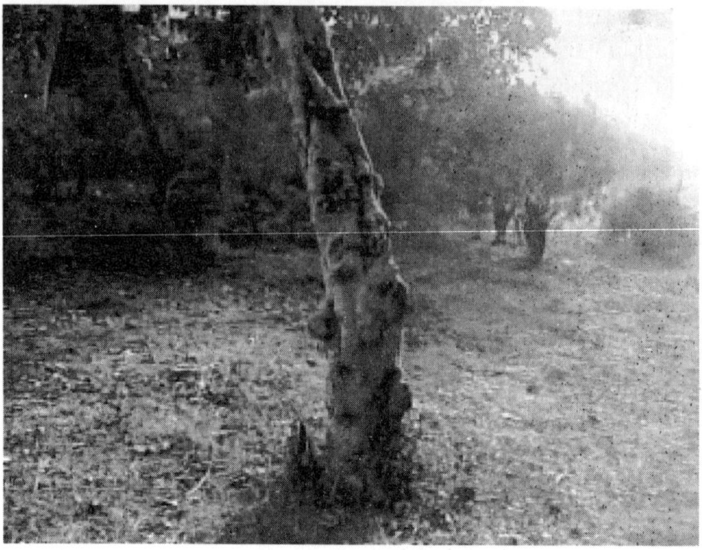

Deformity in Trees

conjunction of high power lines, underground water streams and Hartmann grid crossing should be considered as extreme perturbation of the ambient field. It should be essential to have a correct positioning of beds in places where people have diminished resistance and health such as hospitals. The Earth is an electromagnetic body, with its diminishing method.

At the time of an earthquake, the Hartmann grid is distorted, taking about 30 minutes to resume its former state. In addition, at the more powerful crossing points of this system, there is a 50% increase of radioactivity. He states those twelve hours prior to an earthquake, weak secondary rays can be found, one on each side of the main wave, gathering in strength until they are the same as the central one. There is another much tighter grid pattern called Curry Grid, after a Swiss doctor, Dr. Manfred Curry.

Curry Lines

Curry lines form a global grid network of electrically charged lines of natural origin. These lines runs diagonally North East to South West and South East to North West and were identified by Dr. Manfred Curry and Dr. Wittmann–The distance between the lines is approximately 3 meters (may vary). In Delhi, generally the distance is around 2m. As lines are electrically charged, the intersection points are double positive, double negative or neutral. It has alternate charging and discharging nodes.

If the lines are under the bed, a tremendous discharge of energy will occur from the physical body. This position of the lines can change due to natural vibrations of earth such as earthquakes. Curry lines are called CANCER LINES in Europe. Curry grid has a unusual characteristic of waking the people in the mid night between 1:00 am to 3:00 am as the energy level of body depletes by midnight and body finds a need for rejuvenate itself. The reasons of waking may vary from day to day, person to person or time to time.

Black Lines

Black lines seem to be naturally generated. They may be localized and do not form a network in the same way as Hartmann and Curry lines. Black lines or black streams are more difficult to define. They may be what a Ley line becomes after it passes through a graveyard or they may be produced by a very powerful water flow. EMF's radiating up from subterranean streams, that are polluted by radon, pesticides, or natural minerals will create black streams at the surface. It is a noxious force of natural origin that, like Ley lines, has no set pattern. They can be curved, straight, at ground level or higher.

Black streams can be defined as underground water veins or streams that give off noxious radiations which can be harmful to life above them. They can be conceptualized as earth meridians whose flow has become stagnant or polluted, giving raise to Negative Energy. Harmful radiation rises in a vertical plane from the underground stream to the earth's surface. Black Streams have been found to be anywhere from 1 ft to 900ft deep and from 1ft to 300ft wide.

Black Streams have been known to change their habitual course, especially after earthquakes and droughts. They are known to be stronger at midday, mid-summer, full moon, and during periods of heightened solar flare (sunspot) activity. A black stream is a sick earth meridian. There is a well- established link between black streams and traumas to the earth's etheric web that have caused the flow of energy to stagnate in these channels. Typical examples of such traumas include the building of railway and highway cuttings, tunnels, quarries, mines, and building foundations, especially those with steel footings. Also implicated are heavy industry sites, power stations and electricity sub-stations, military bases, steel pilings, poles and even road signs. Old battle grounds and historical sites involving trauma to the earth or to humans, such as witch-burning sites, execution grounds, and burial grounds can also retain much negativities. Sometimes natural topography can exhibit similar effects, particularly if there are concentrations of iron ore below ground. A person can suffer from Heart problem, Slip-disk or Hernia if sleeping for long time exactly on the top of powerful geopathic stress and black streams.

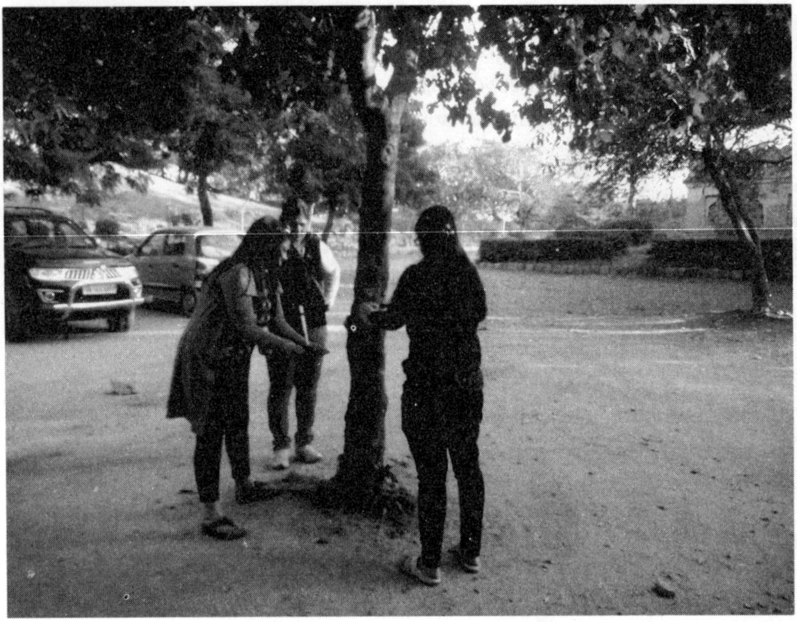

Geobiological Detection

Ley Lines

Ley lines are alignments of ancient sites stretching across the landscape. Ancient sites or holy places may be situated in a straight line ranging from one or two to several miles in length. Ley lines are generally recognized as man-made phenomena, occurring where sacred stones which have been charged energetically, naturally and spontaneously, if at least 5 such stones are placed in line within a distance of 25 miles. These lines are found at most ancient monuments and sacred places along the water lines. Many ancient sites can be connected to form an incredible coincidence of interconnecting lines.

A power centre is created by the presence of both ley energy and underground water. The combination of the two creates a power that has the capability to not only affect consciousness, but also to retain the feelings of people. The average length of a ley line is twenty to thirty miles, although the length can vary from only a few feet to thousands of miles. The average width of the ley line can be up to 2m.

Symptoms Associated with Geopathic Stress

1. Weak Immune System
2. Sleeping disorders and Nightmares
3. Disorders like Sweating, Freezing

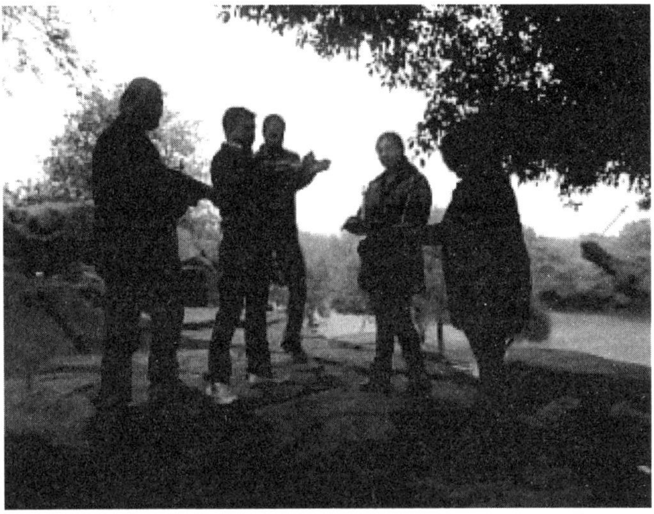

Detecting Ley Lines

4. Migraines, Tensions, Headaches
5. Difficult to Concentrate
6. Persistence of any symptoms despite treatments
7. Skin problems-Itching and Eczema
8. Cancer
9. Feeling tired in the morning
10. Long-term stress in relationships/work
11. You feel healthier when you are away from home
12. Previous occupants suffered serious illness
13. Lack of growth in plants
14. Schizophrenia
15. Short-term memory loss

It is said that when we are spending our 1/3 of life on bed that is 8 hours, the positioning is very important at night. When we are asleep; our subconscious mind is highly active. We need to get repaired by ourselves while we are asleep. Geopathic stress continuously affects our body for 6 to 8 hours during sleep. A vulnerable individual exposed to the negative influence of Geopathic radiations for a prolonged period of time on a static position. Genetically inherited weaknesses manifest themselves in the form of diseases. This is determined by the degree of radiation's intensity and the length of exposure, to the Geopathic stress. Geopathic stress or poor quality land is fairly a big factor contributing to Sick Building Syndrome.

Small babies, unable to move away, may react to a zone of disturbance by showing signs of slow development, prolonged crying, convulsive crying or screaming. Young children, able to move, will instinctively flee from zones of disturbance. They may be found sleeping on the floor, another bed or on a chair, or, if they cannot escape from a crib, they may be found crouched or curled up in one of the corners. Children, able to talk, may tell of a presence in their bed, or show signs of fear that someone or something is in their room. Children are very sensitive where there is a spot or section of geopathy, they avoid going there or sleep there, and they show their strong opposition to enter the section or spot.

Indicators of Zones in the Bedroom

We spend a considerable time in bed. Six to nine hours a night and sleep in basically one general area; it is wise to be aware of symptoms that can arise through the presence of zones of disturbance.

1. Refusal to go to bed. Opposition against going to bed.
2. Insomnia. Unable to fall asleep for hours.
3. Nightmares. Feelings of a "presence" in the bed.
4. An aversion to certain spots in the bed.
5. A feeling of "falling out" of bed.
6. Night sweats. Also feeling cold or shivering in bed.
7. Waking up tired most mornings; fatigue.
8. Nausea in the morning, even vomiting.
9. Stress, depression.
10. Frequent crying upon waking up in the morning.
11. Rapid heart beat while lying still in bed; cramps.

Naturally, one of these symptoms is sufficient to indicate a problem. However, there may be several of these symptoms appearing at one time. When you are sensitive to Geopathic stress and sleep away from home in a non-geopathically stressed area, you will probably find that you sleep better and feel more energized.

Various effects of Earth's (naturally occurring or man-made) unhealthy energies can be found:

1. Directly above an underground 'unhealthy' river or stream
2. Downstream of two graveyards
3. Downstream of a quarry. (In a working quarry, this depends on the type of rock being quarried, whether dynamite is or has been used, and the amount of dust emitted. On the site of an old graveyard or battlefield

4. Wells radiating into an energy ley passing through a cemetery, refuse or chemical dump, etc. (Wells are usually sited on crossing underground streams). In addition, sometimes disused wells are pressed into service as septic tanks.
5. Above and around deep coal mines, especially if they are disused and flooded
6. Other old mine workings
7. Ionizing radiation from radioactive contaminations.
8. The area close to power cables near quarries and geological faults
9. The area near busy railway lines. This only extends to about 40 meters on unelectrified tracks, but very much further downstream of electrified lines
10. Around transformers and turbines at power stations
11. Around nuclear reactors and dumps, missile storage sites
12. Above underground train systems
13. Crossing energy leys from standing stones and circles
14. On the downstream side of banks of polluted rivers, canals
15. Vibrations from exobiological faults and its fractures
16. Vibrations due to friction from the movement of underground water through rock strata
17. Underground caves, tunnels, mines
18. Battle fields, buried ground, massacre sites
19. Virtually any place where traumatic emotional event has occurred
20. Landfill sites where material have been buried such as metal objects, garbage, pollutants
21. Roads- railways tracks, power lines, cables, switch boards, TVs and computers or mobiles.

Accident Prone Areas on the Road

A statically puzzling reality is that road accidents happen more often at specific locations on the roads or highways that don't look particularly dangerous. The study of such spots can reveal the reports of noticing congestion in these road sections. A place on road where repetitive accidents happen frequently may indicate geopathic stress. In our day today life we can notice such local points in every city. Some of our students have done extensive research on roads and geopathic stress.

The vehicle normally runs at a speed of 60 kms. per hour or 15 meters per second. It means the vehicle crosses the road boundaries if the brain fails to communicate even for two Seconds, (30 meters). The vehicle will be out of the road causing accident. The driver always gives priority on time and speed to reach his destiny. In this regard, he vibrates in different frequencies, sometimes these negative frequencies clashes with the positive brain frequencies, of the drive, this obstructs the process of the brain waves in their communication power ever for two three seconds causing dreadful accidents.

The brain is normally weighting 700gm to 1 kg approximately, which possesses ten billion neurons (cells approximately). That the Earth is vibrates at a frequency of 7.5 to 14 htz., (Alpha Level). But the human brain about more or less above the frequency as they are driving with attention. The brain frequency may vary depending upon temperament and character of the person. Due to presence of Geopathic stress on Highways, the earth at that spot may vibrate above 200 htz. Which is not acceptable and Digestible to the brain waves.

These neurons are capable of communicating to the other cells in the body to the tune of 1 lakh per second with other parts of the body namely eyes, legs and hand etc. or any system of the body during driving. If this communication system fails due to negative radiations, (frequencies less than400nm and above 700nm) even for 2 or 3 seconds, the vehicle will be out of the road causing accidents. In nature the voids of energy soil are partly or completely filled with water. The water may be in a state of rest or in a state of flow. If it is in a state of rest, the method for solving stability and deformation problems are essentially identical with those solving similar problems.

Rectifications and Remedies for Geopathic Stress

It is very important to have synergy between human energy and Earth energy to live life happily. It means one should be very cautious where the house, work place, is and the energy is balanced with him to avoid unnecessary troubles. Nowadays, in the whole world, people are aware of Ecology and balancing them with Earth's energies. People are now using natural building materials and follow Green concepts for healthy living.

The most effective way of dealing with geopathic stress is to move one's bed and other pieces of furniture. Once the geopathic stress lines have been identified, the simple measure of **moving out of the area of geopathic stress** often solves the problem. The further the bed can be moved the more likely it is that one gets out of the stressed area. For some, it is impossible to move their bed and in this case other methods need to be tried. Architects and Interior Designers must plan the furniture layout considering the geological conditions of the building.

The second best solution of Geopathic stress is **changing the soil** and getting fertile soil placed in the geopathically stressed land. In this case soil test is essential to proceed.

In certain cases, there may be a grid pattern of unhealthy waves present at intersections with a bed, and it is not practicable to move the bed to any safer location. In order to reduce the negativity of stress, we can use raw sea salt; basil leaves powder or Panchgavya to clear the negative energies from the land, as per requirement. It may be possible to diminish the harm of stress by planting genus buxus above the place.

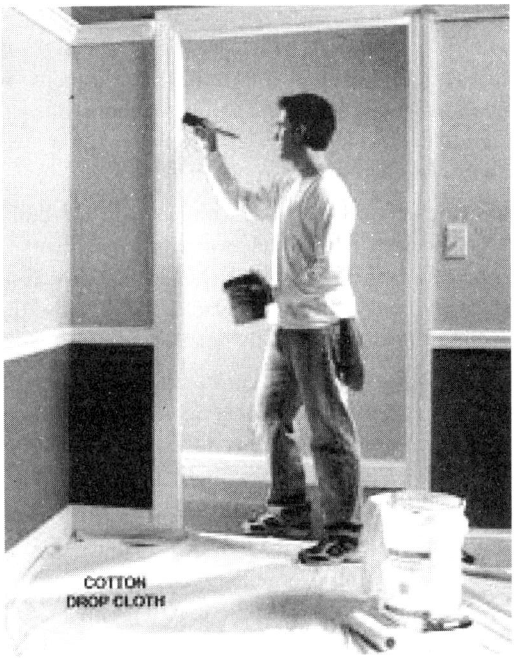

Chemical Sensitivity from Paints

Building Materials and Multiple Chemical Sensitivity

Science & technology have been advancing at a phenomenal peace in recent times. The day to day discoveries & innovations are fast reaching every household the world over, greatly affecting over life-style. An understanding of basic materials used in the manufacture of various household articles equips the home makers with necessary knowledge to make effective decision choices from the infinite range of materials available. In order to put this material to their optimal use & be able to maintain them properly, it is very important to know their chemistry; i.e. their composition and properties. This is a difficult area to address in one paragraph, but great care should be given to what materials are used and how they are used. The danger lies in not just what makes up a material, but in how it is used. Always prefer healthy building materials for self and client.

Wise Selection of Building Materials

Various type of building materials are available in the market. The designers need to consider architectural and interior related material after considering the broad technical literature of the product. Every building material has its own characteristics. The various characteristics should therefore be considered before choosing them. Some of the factors to be kept in mind are-.

a. **Local Availability**–Materials which are locally available suit the climatic conditions. They generally suit the overall environment. Such materials help in conservation of energy and hence reduction of cost. For example Agra red is a stone which can suit anywhere but it would have best suitability with the climate in Agra itself.

b. **Ecological Impact**–The ecological impact of the building material should be considered. For instance asbestos has been considered, as the contaminating building material, therefore it should not be used. If in case, asbestos is used, special contractors who know the way to deal asbestos whiling, cutting or demolishing should be considered.

c. **Energy Consumption**–Before considering any building material, check the energy consumption. Energy conservation is important, good conductors generally transfer energy faster and at a higher rate while insulators are poor conductor of heat, light and energy. Insulators should be preferred in comparison to conductors in case of energy consumption.

d. **Out gassing**–There are building materials available which outgas harmful chemicals. These chemicals can be dangerous and create serious diseases for the user. For example combustible material emits CO, which is very harmful for human body.

e. **Natural Occurrence**–Before purchasing building material one must prioritize materials having natural occurrences for example solid wood should be preferred in comparison to pressed woods like block board, particle board or MDF. Natural stone should be preferred in comparison to any artificial material preferred.

f. **Diffusion & breathing**–The building material opted should be capable of breathing. The air and energy circulation should not stop. There are various material which act as a complete blockage and such material should not be considered.

g. **Hygroscopicity**–Hygroscopicity is the quality of material to absorb and hold water. The level of hygroscopicity should also be considered before purchasing it. It should be made sure that the material has hygroscopicity.

h. **Fire Retardani & Termite Proof**- Prefer those building materials which are termite proof and fire retardant. They would ensure safety at users end.

Other than the above mentioned characteristics. Capacity to absorb toxic vapours and gases, sound transmission, Heat storage capacity, Resistance to electrostatic charges, surface temperature and conductivity should also be considered. The building materials we use, our building practices, and attitudes to technology and science need reconsideration, and for all natural systems. Natural hygroscope (breathing) building materials absorb and release moisture readily; filtering out air pollution and releasing clear air in the transaction. Such materials should replace mechanical ventilation and air conditioning. Chemicals from nature should replace those synthesized by science. Building should be sited with an understanding of natural terrestrial radiation so that areas affected by ionized radiation can be avoided.

Sites and building materials need to be chosen according to how well they minimize stress from noise. Planning of settlements should integrate low density housing with open space bar recreation, perm culture, indigenous vegetation, shelter belts, areas of companion planting, and areas devoted to fish and livestock. All building products should be in connect with building biology and human ecology. The bioclimate affects human and well-being. We would be discussing the triggers to health through building materials later in the chapter. Lets understand how human body responds sensitively to chemical emissions from building materials and how multiple chemical sensitivity can lead to Sick Building Syndrome.

Multiple Chemical Sensitivity

Multiple Chemical Sensitivity; in broad terms means an unusually severe sensitivity or allergy-like reaction to many different kinds of pollutants including solvents, VOC's (Volatile Organic Compounds), perfumes, petrol, diesel, smoke, "chemicals" in general and often encompasses problems with regard to pollen, house dust mites, and pet fur & dander etc. The avoidance of pollutants or toxicants is the key.

The Symptoms of Multiple Chemical Sensitivity

The possible list of symptoms of Multiple Chemical Sensitivity is almost endless - varies from one patient to another. Most sufferers of MCS complain of at least several of the following:

- Extreme Fatigue/Lethargy
- Headache/Migraine/Vertigo/Dizziness
- Poor memory and concentration

Burning Eyes

- Burning, stinging eyes
- Wheezing, breathlessness, nausea

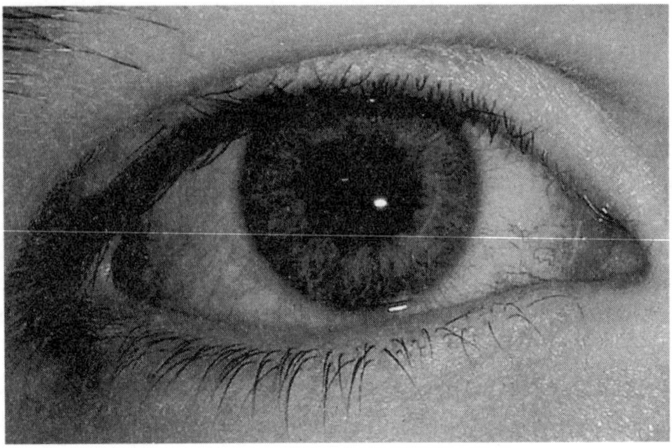

- Runny nose (Rhinitis)
- Sore throat, cough
- Sinus problems

Skin Rashes

- Skin rashes and/or itching skin
- Sensitivity to light & noise

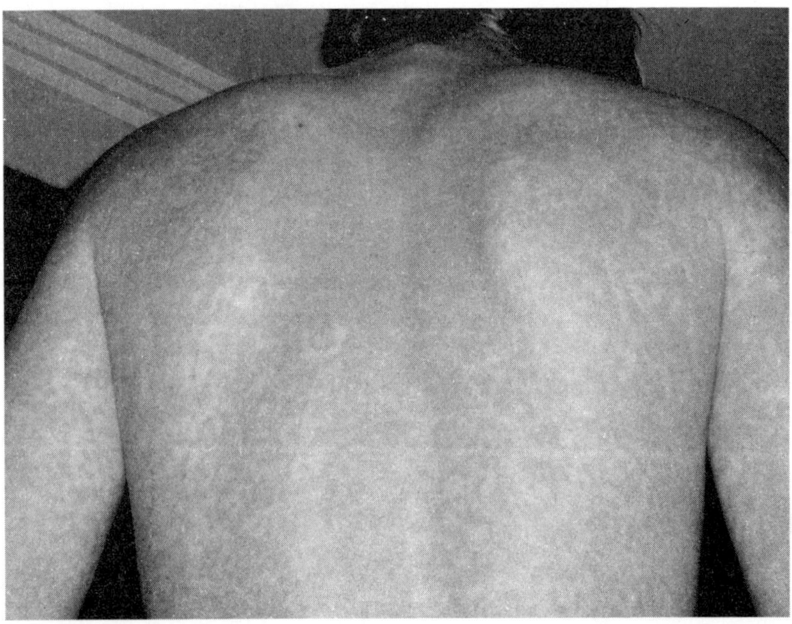

- Sleeping problems
- Immune system disorders
- Digestive upset, and
- Muscle and joint pain.

Enzyme Depletion

Detoxification of all manner of naturally occurring toxins is carried out in humans by enzymes in the liver. These same enzymes are also used to detoxify a wide range of synthetic chemicals, but, if the enzymes are depleted or damaged by health problems, then they are unable to metabolize these toxicants efficiently, so leading to the problems associated with Multiple Chemical Sensitivity.

Enzyme depletion is used to great effect with some types of pesticide, where the action of the primary poison is augmented by the use of an enzyme blocker so that the poison cannot be metabolized properly, remains in the body of the organism longer, and so is much more highly toxic than it would otherwise be. Many types of enzyme deficiency can be inherited & this may

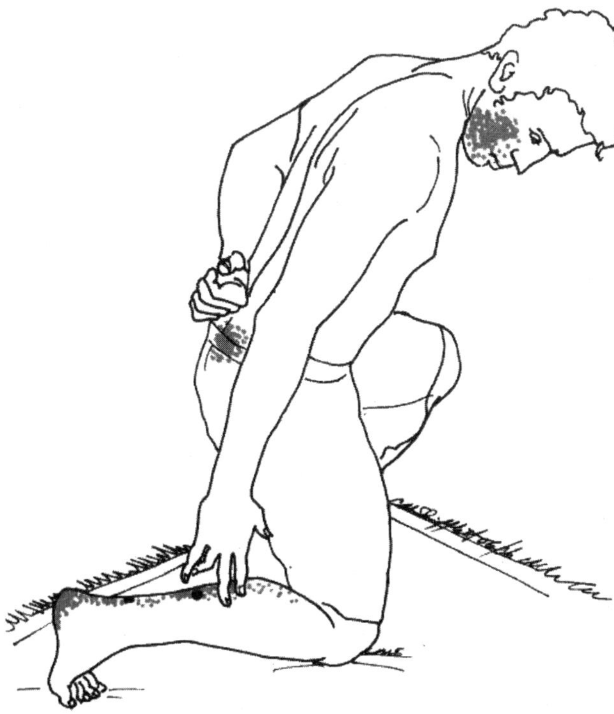

Joint Pain

lead one to suppose that MCS may affect other members of the same family and, in fact, there is some (fairly tentative) evidence to support this view.

Immune System Damage

Some researchers are of the opinion that Multiple Chemical Sensitivity is due to immune system damage or malfunction, which could give rise to sensitivity to all sorts of triggers rather than a specific reaction to one toxicant.

A number of types of toxic chemicals have been implicated in major single exposures for people who then subsequently became MCS sufferers and which are known to be Immune System disruptors; these include *organochlorines, formaldehyde, pesticides, herbicides, organophosphates* and others.

Another important and debilitating feature of MCS - and which tends to complicate MCS diagnosis & treatment still further - is it's ability to apparently augment the effects of other problems experienced by the patient - problems such as *common allergies, asthma, depression, food intolerances* etc, and these problems of *augmentation* are reported by about *half* of all MCS sufferers.

The Environmental Illness Resource says Multiple Chemical Sensitivity is the name given to a syndrome in which a sufferer experiences multiple symptoms upon exposure to minute amounts of everyday chemicals. There is currently no officially recognized definition for Multiple Chemical Sensitivity. This is due to the fact that very little is known about it, especially the mechanisms involved with the onset of symptoms. A couple of theories suggest a possible role for a hypersensitive central nervous system, immune dysfunction and impaired detoxification by liver enzymes.

Triggers–Unhealthy Building Materials

Reactions in MCS are triggered by a vast array of everyday chemicals from perfume to diesel exhaust. The common ingredients in most of these chemical products are hydrocarbon based volatile organic chemicals (VOC's). Phenols (containing benzene) are commonly implicated. With everyday cosmetic and household chemical products, it is generally the addition of perfume that makes them bad news for MCS sufferers. Typically a sufferer will notice a sensitivity to one or two things to start with, perfume and cigarette smoke for example, and then will rapidly become sensitized to more and more chemical sources over a relatively short period of time. The reasons for this common occurrence are unknown but it is clearly something that needs to be investigated.

Common chemical triggers of Multiple Chemical Sensitivity as per Environmental illness Resource are:

New Carpet

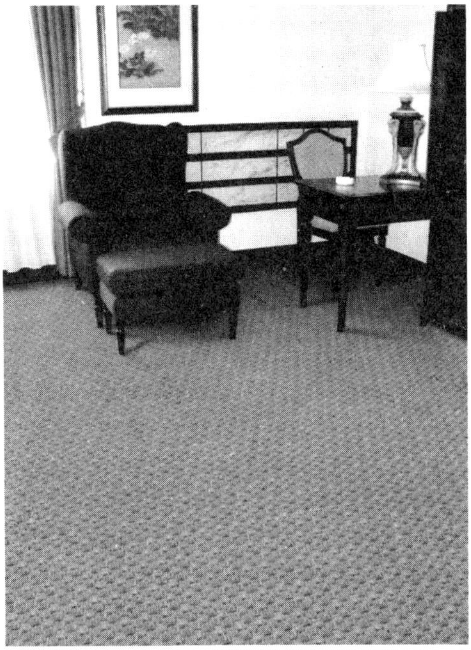

Off Gas from Carpets

Most new carpets contain a cocktail of volatile organic compounds (VOC's) as ingredients in glues, backing materials, flame retardants, dyes etc. These include many of the chemicals we are now familiar with, such as acetone, toluene, xylene, formaldehyde, and benzene derivatives. When the carpet is new these chemicals "off gas" over a period of around 6 months to 2 years, polluting the air in the home.

Lead and VOC Paints

Paint which emits Volatile Organic Compounds are dangerous for human health. Considering the negative aspect of VOC emission, Green Building guidelines emphasize on VOC free paints to be used in buildings.

Particle Board

Manufactured particle board is now used much more widely than solid wood in our homes, in such things as fitted kitchens, furniture such as shelving, bookcases, cabinets (especially flat-pack) and laminate flooring. Particle board is basically wood chip bound together by chemical adhesives into solid boards. As with new carpets, new particle board products off gas VOC's over a relatively long period of time and will trigger symptoms in the chemically sensitive and may induce sensitivity in previously healthy individuals. Chemicals that off gas from particle board are similar to those from carpets with **formaldehyde** most often the main offender.

CCA-treated Timber

CCA treated timber contains a mixture of chemical compounds containing copper, chromium and arsenic. It is a preservative used to treat wood to stop it rotting when used outdoors. CCA treated timber was developed in the 1930s and has been used ever since. It is a potential health risk as it contains arsenic. Children are most likely to be at risk through biting or eating timber in structures such as playgrounds, sandpit surrounds and decks.

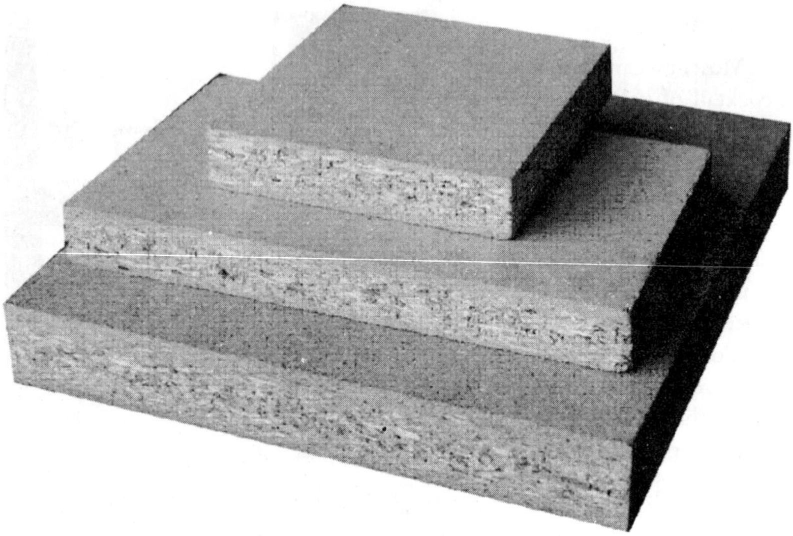

Formaldehyde Emissions

PCBs

Polychlorinated biphenyls (PCBs) are a group of over 200 chemicals which were commonly used in fluorescent tubes and other electrical equipment made before 1980. These substances are highly toxic and do not break down quickly. Between 1994 and 1998 there was a nation-wide programme to identify and dispose of any fittings and equipment containing PCBs.

Plastics

All of the petrochemical-based materials in use today share a common legacy of emitting toxic chemicals in the process of refining the oil or gas from which these plastics are made. Chlorinated plastics, including polyvinyl chloride, however, have come under more intense scrutiny due to the extreme toxicity of chemicals involved in their production and disposal.

Why Are Chlorinated Plastics a Problem?

Throughout the lifecycle of PVC and other chlorinated plastics, through manufacture and disposal, the chlorine content has the potential to produce dioxins. Dioxins are an unavoidable by-product of the manufacture, combustion, and disposal of materials containing chlorine, which can create dioxins both when the products are manufactured and when they burn in structural fibres or at the end of their useful life in incinerators or landfill fibres. Dioxins include some of the most potent carcinogens known to humankind. One of the most toxic dioxin compounds is not only a carcinogen, but also a reproductive and developmental toxicant and alters the immune and endocrine systems. Dioxins are a family of compounds widely recognized as persistent bioaccumulative toxicants (PBTs), which has led to them becoming a global problem. The US Green Building Council has acknowledged that the chlorine content of PVC building materials and the resultant dioxin emissions "puts PVC consistently among the **worst materials for human health** impacts.

Asbestos

Asbestos is a substance found in certain building products. These products include:

- Asbestos cement cladding
- Textured ceiling coatings
- Thermal insulation around pipes, and
- Boilers fire-protective linings on structural steel (limpet asbestos).

Asbestos can cause lung disease with sufficient exposure.

Perfume

According to a 1986 report by the Committee on Science & Technology, U.S. House of Representatives, 95% of chemicals in perfumes and fragrance

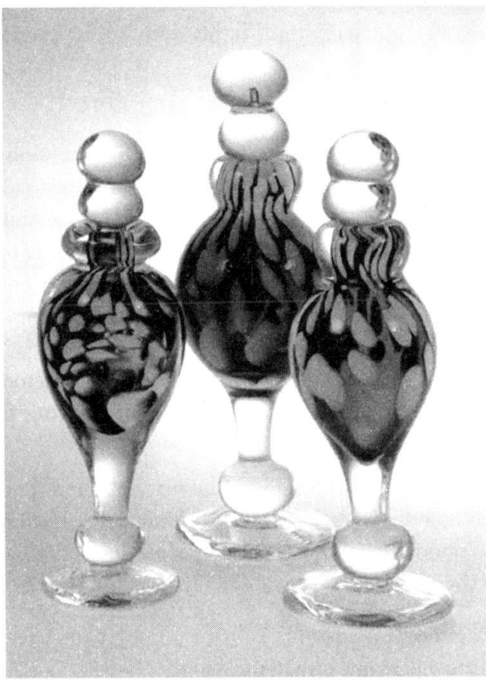

Perfumes can be Contaminating

products are synthetic chemicals derived from petroleum. Some of the major perfume ingredients include benzaldehyde, benzyl acetate, benzyl alcohol, ethanol, ethyl acetate, limonene, linalool, a-pinene, g-terpinene and a-terpineol. All of these chemicals are known to have negative health consequences, mainly due to effects on the central nervous system.

Household Cleaning Products

The Environmental Protection Agency (EPA) in the US states that the air in the average home may be up to 5 times as polluted as the air outside. Much of this pollution comes from the use of common household cleaning products. They also caution that of the many thousands of chemicals in use only around 3 in 10 have actually been safety tested. Examples of common chemicals in cleaning products include diethyl phthalate, found in a range of products, toluene, found in stain removers, and hexane/xylene, found in aerosol sprays. Diethyl Phthalate is a known endocrine disrupter (interferes with hormone activity), toluene is a known carcinogen (cancer causing agent) and can cause neurological problems, and finally both hexane and xylene can also damage the nervous system.

Other cleaning products that commonly trigger MCS symptoms include dishwasher detergent, laundry liquid/powder, fabric softener, air "fresheners", and bathroom/kitchen detergents. Highly fragranced products are always likely to be the most troublesome.

Personal Care Products and Cosmetics

Equally important contributors to indoor air pollution are the many personal care and cosmetic products that fill bathroom cabinets etc. The added danger with many of these, such as hair spray and deodorant, is that we carry the chemicals around with us all day on our bodies. Some of the common chemicals found in such products include cocoamide DEA (detergent in most shampoos, moisturisers and more), propylene glycol (in deodorant, shampoos, shaving gels, moisturisers and more), sodium lauryl sulphate (detergents- in shampoos, toothpastes, more), acetone (nail varnish remover) and benzaldehyde (hair spray, deodorant, shaving foam, shampoo, bar soap and more).

Other problem products include shower gels and liquid soaps, nail varnish, hair styling products, hair conditioners, sun lotion, and scented bath products. Again the highly fragranced products tend to be the most troublesome to the multiple chemical sensitivity patient.

Other common triggers:

The above is by no means an exhaustive list. Here are some other common triggers of symptoms in MCS patients:

- Marker pens
- Soft plastics
- New clothes
- New furniture
- Newspapers/magazines
- Paint
- Varnish
- Solvents
- Glues/adhesives, and more

The Impact of Multiple Chemical Sensitivity on Quality of Life

Multiple Chemical Sensitivity is a devastating illness, not just because of the distress caused by the symptoms themselves, but also from the resulting effects on all areas of life. An MCS sufferer typically becomes more and more isolated and withdrawn as they simply can't be around people (wearing perfume, deodorant etc) or in public spaces where chemicals are routinely used. MCS sufferers often lose their jobs as they can't tolerate the chemicals in the work environment, and relationships often break down as the partner is unable to understand or adapt to living without the use of common chemical products.

Immune System

A couple of studies have found abnormal T and B-lymphocyte numbers and increased auto antibodies, that is antibodies that react with the body's own tissues. Some data has shown a low T-helper/Suppressor ratio which would act to impair immune function. Probably the most consistent finding is that of low natural killer (NK) cell activity. This is interesting in the light of strong evidence for low NK activity in chronic fatigue syndrome and fibromyalgia. The inconsistent findings have been suggested to be the result of changes in immune activation over time following an exposure, with the resulting difficulties in testing MCS patients appropriately in research studies.

Pollutant	Sources	Effects on Humans
Benzene: A commonly used solvent, also found in fuels.	Inks, oils, paints, plastics, rubber, gasoline, detergents, pharmaceuticals, dyes, tobacco smoke and synthetic fibres.	Skin and eye irritation (including drying, inflammation, blistering and dermatitis), dizziness, weakness, headache, nausea, blurred vision, respiratory problems, tremors, irregular heartbeat, liver and kidney damage, loss of appetite, drowsiness, nervousness, psychological disturbances, diseases of the blood system and carcinogenicity.

Pollutant	Sources	Effects on Humans
Formaldehyde: A disinfectant, preservative, and curing agent.	Particle board, pressed wood, foam insulation, paper bags, waxed papers, facial tissues, stiffeners and wrinkle resisters, water repellents, fire retardants, binders in floor coverings, carpet backing, permanent press clothes, natural gas, kerosene and cigarette smoke.	Irritation of mucous membranes of the eyes, nose and throat, allergic contact dermatitis, respiratory problems, eye irritation, headaches, asthma and carcinogenicity to the throat.
Trichloroethylene: A commercial product for industrial use.	Metal degreasers, dry cleaners, printing inks, lacquers, varnishes and adhesives.	Potent carcinogenicity to the liver.

How Plants Clean Air

Plants have proven to be important life supporters in that they remove carbon dioxide from the air and release oxygen through the process of photosynthesis. The NASA studies found that plants also work in a symbiotic relationship to remove air pollutants produced by other plants, people and industry. Trace chemicals in the atmosphere are absorbed and biodegraded by plant leaves and roots, the soil, and micro-organisms. Virtually every tropical foliage and flowering plant works to remove pollutants from the interior environment, and particular plants are better at removing certain toxins. The studies found that one potted plant per 100 square feet of floor space can help clean the air in the average home or office, although the addition of more plants would increase the rate of pollutant removal.

Air Purifying Plants

The following list of plants typically used in the interior environment outlines the plants found to be most effective in air purification, based on the NASA studies.

Plant Name	Toxins Removed
Aechmea fasciata Bromeliad	Excellent for formaldehyde and xylene
Aglaonema modestum Chinese Evergreen	Excellent for benzene and toluene

Plant Name	Toxins Removed
Aloe vera Aloe	Excellent for formaldehyde
Chamaedorea seifrizii Bamboo Palm	Excellent for benzene and formaldehyde
Chlorophytum elatum Spider Plant	Excellent for carbon monoxide and formaldehyde
Chrysanthemum morifolium Pot Mum	Excellent for trichloroethylene, good for benzene and formaldehyde
Dendrobium Orchid	Excellent for acetone, ammonia, chloroform, ethyl acetate, methyl alcohol, formaldehyde and xylene
Dieffenbachia maculata Dumbcane	Good for formaldehyde
Dracaena deremensis "Janet Craig" Janet Craig	Excellent for benzene and trichloroethylene.
Dracaena deremensis "Warneckii" Warneckii	Excellent for benzene and trichloroethylene, good for formaldehyde
Dracaena marginata Madagascar Dragon Tree	Excellent for benzene, good for formaldehyde and trichloroethylene
Dracaena massangeana Mass Cane	Excellent for formaldehyde
Epipremnum aureum Golden Pothos	Excellent for carbon monoxide and benzene, good for formaldehyde
Euphorbia pulcherima Poinsettia	Excellent for formaldehyde
Ficus benjamina Weeping Fig	Good for formaldehyde
Gerbera jamesonii Gerbera Daisy	Excellent for benzene and trichloroethylene, good for formaldehyde
Guzmania "Cherry" Bromeliad	Excellent for formaldehyde and xylene
Hedera helix English Ivy	Excellent for benzene, good for formaldehyde and trichloroethylene

Plant Name	Toxins Removed
Liriope muscari "Variegata" Variegated Lily-turf	Excellent for formaldehyde
Musa oriana Banana	Excellent for formaldehyde
Neoregelia carolinae "Perfecta Tricolor" Bromeliad	Good for xylene
Peperomia obtusifolia Peperomia	Good for formaldehyde
Phalaenopsis Orchid	Excellent for formaldehyde and xylene
Philodendron domesticum Elephant Ear Philodendron	Excellent for formaldehyde
Philodendron oxycardium Heart Leaf Philodendron	Excellent for formaldehyde
Philodendron selloum Lacy Tree Philodenron	Excellent for formaldehyde
Rhododendron indicum Azalea	Good for formaldehyde
Sansevieria trifasciata "Laurentii" Mother-in-law's Tongue	Excellent for benzene and formaldehyde, good for trichloroethylene
Schefflera arboricola Miniature Umbrella Plant	Good for benzene, formaldehyde and toluene
Spathiphyllum "Mauna Loa" Peace Lily	Excellent for benzene and trichloroethylene, good for formaldehyde
Syngonium podophyllum Arrowhead Plant	Good for formaldehyde
Tradescantia sillamontana Oyster Plant	Good for formaldehyde

Indoor Air Quality and Sick Building Syndrome

Indoor Air has an immense impact on our health. It is considered to be one of the most important reasons for creation of Sick Building Syndrome in a building. The U.S. Environmental Protection Agency (EPA) highlights that indoor air pollutant levels are much more than outdoor levels. It is observed that people spent most of their time indoors and therefore they are prone to risk existing due to poor indoor air quality. The below mentioned problems are arising due to such indoor air pollution:

- *Reducedperformanceandefficiencylevelsofoccupantsduetodiscomfort,sickness,or absenteeism*
- *Increasing deterioration of the building and inefficiency of the equipment within the structure.*
- *Strained relationships due to irritability, fatigue, stress, pressures and aggressions among the staff in office, labour in factory and occupants in a home.*
- *Increase in short term and long term health problems for occupants.*

Indoor air problems can sometimes be subtle and do not always produce easily recognizable impacts on health. Children may be especially susceptible to air pollution. Indoor air quality is of high concern these days and proper maintenance of indoor air is more than a "quality" issue as it encompasses health and safety.

Over the past several years, the construction of more tightly sealed buildings, reduced ventilation rates to save energy, the use of synthetic building materials and furnishings have highly increased. The use of chemically-formulated personal care products, pesticides, and housekeeping supplies have also gone up. All these factors have highly contributed to poor indoor air quality and the need for environmentally friendly solutions which should be both holistic and scientific.

Sources of Indoor Air Pollution

Indoor air contaminants can originate within the building or from outdoors. Air pollutants consist of numerous particulates, fibres, mists, bio-acrosols, and gases. Another important aspect of indoor air pollution is that it can vary by time and location within the facilities, or even a single room. Pollutants can be emitted from recognizable point sources, such as from chemical store rooms, or from area sources, such as newly painted surfaces.

Typical Sources of Indoor Air Pollutants include:

Outdoor Air Pollution

- Pollen
- Dust
- Fungal spores
- Industrials emissions
- Vehicle emissions
- Unsanitary debris or building exhausts near outdoor air intakes
- Loading docks
- Odours from dumpsters

- Underground Sources
- Radon emission
- Pesticides
- Leakage from underground storage tanks

HVAC Equipment

- Microbiological growth in drip pans, ductwork, coils, and humidifiers
- Improper venting of combustion products
- Dust or debris in ductwork

Non-HVAC Equipment

- Emissions from office equipment (volatile organic compounds)
- Emissions from shops, labs, cleaning processes

Components

- Microbiological growth on soiled or water-damaged materials
- Dry traps that allow the passage of sewer gas
- Materials containing volatile organic compounds, inorganic compounds or asbestos
- Materials that produce particles (dust)

Miscellaneous

- Emissions from new furnishings and floorings
- Microbiological growth on or in soiled or water-damaged furnishings
- Science laboratories
- Copy/print areas
- Food prep areas
- Smoking lounges
- Cleaning materials
- Personal care products
- Emissions from trash
- Pesticides
- Odours and volatile organic compounds from paint, chalk, adhesives
- Occupants with communicable diseases
- Dry-erase markers and similar pens
- Insects and other pests

Other Indoor Air Contaminants

There are a variety of sources and factors that can contribute to the cause and spread of IAQ contaminants. These sources may result in a variety of IAQ contaminants including:

- Radon
- Environmental Tobacco Smoke

- Biological Contaminants (mold, mildew, etc.)
- Stoves, Heaters, Fireplaces, and Chimneys
- Household Products
- Formaldehyde
- Pesticides
- Asbestos
- Lead

Biological Contaminants

Biological contaminants include bacteria, molds, mildew, viruses, animal dander and cat saliva, house dust mites, cockroaches, and pollen. There are many sources of these pollutants. Pollens originate from plants; viruses are transmitted by people and animals; bacteria are carried by people, animals, and soil and plant debris; and household pets are sources of saliva and animal dander. The protein in urine from rats and mice is a potent allergen. When it dries, it can become airborne. Contaminated central air handling systems can become breeding grounds for mold, mildew, and other sources of biological contaminants and can then distribute these contaminants through the home.

By controlling the relative humidity level in a home, the growth of some sources of biological contaminants can be minimized. A relative humidity of 30-50 percent is generally recommended for homes. In any case if the

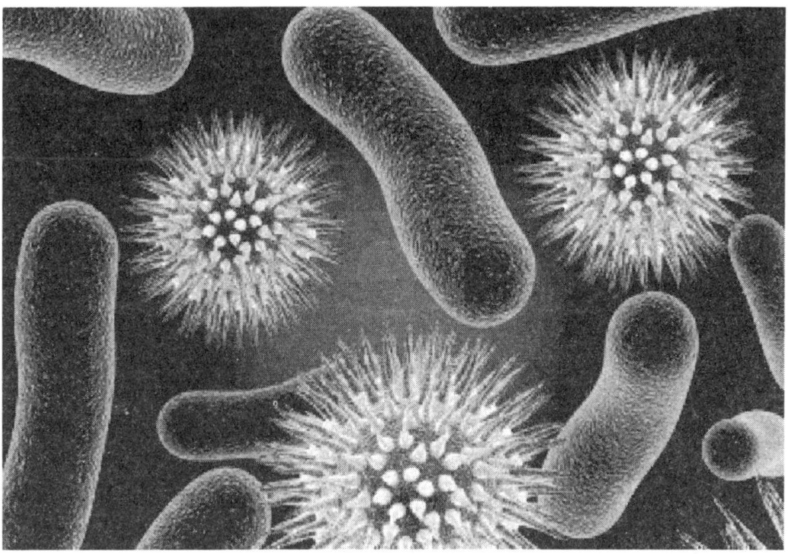

Bacteria

relative humidity goes beyond 70%, it can be lead to organic contaminants. Standing water, water-damaged materials, or wet surfaces also serve as a breeding ground for molds, mildews, bacteria, and insects. House dust mites, the source of one of the most powerful biological allergens, grow in damp, warm environments.

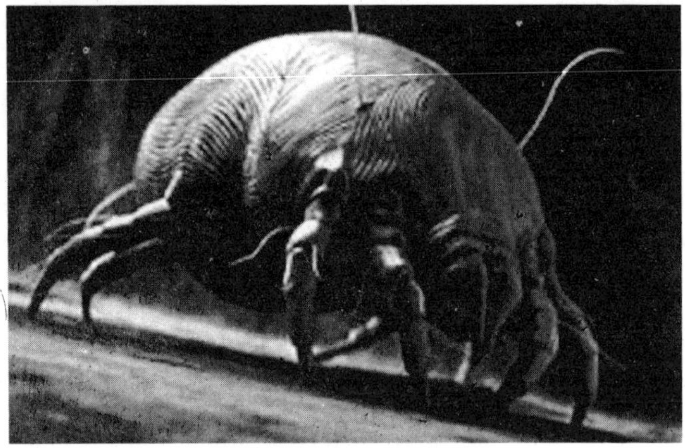

Dustmite

Health Effects from Biological Contaminants:

Some biological contaminants trigger allergic reactions, including hypersensitivity pneumonitis, allergic rhinitis, and some types of asthma. Infectious illnesses, such as influenza, measles, and chicken pox are transmitted through the air. Molds and mildews release disease-causing toxins. Symptoms of health' problems caused by biological pollutants include

- Sneezing,
- Watery eyes,
- Coughing,
- Shortness of breath,
- Dizziness,
- Lethargy,
- Fever, and
- Digestive problems.

Allergic reactions occur generally after repeated exposure to a specific biological allergen. However that reaction may occur immediately upon re-exposure or after multiple exposures over time. As a result, people who have noticed only mild allergic reactions or no reactions may find themselves very sensitive to particular allergens.

Some diseases, like humidifier fever, are associated with exposure to toxins from micro-organisms that can grow in large building ventilation systems. However, these diseases can also be traced to micro-organisms that grow in home heating and cooling systems and humidifiers. Children, elderly people, and people with breathing problems, allergies, and lung diseases are particularly susceptible to disease-causing biological agents in the indoor air.

Mold, Mildew and Other IAQ Contaminants

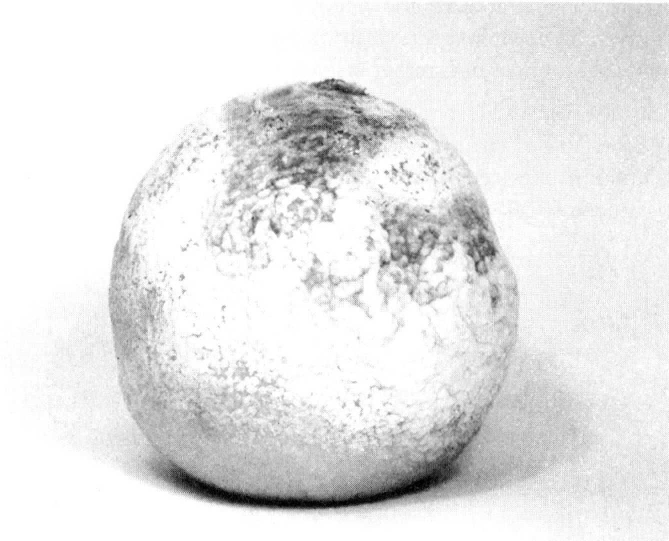

Mold

As discussed earlier high relative humidity is one of the main reasons of growth of mold and mildew. There are variety of sources and factors that can contribute to the cause and spread of indoor air contaminants. Mold is a fungus. We breathe mold spores every day. Molds are part of the natural environment. Molds play an important part in nature by breaking down dead organic matter such as fallen leaves and dead trees. However, indoor mold growth should be avoided. Mold is a growing organism. It produces a "tree-like" structure. At the top of the structure is a "pod". This pod produces the spores which settle out and grow to continue the cycle. When molds produce spores; the millions of tiny spores are invisible to the naked eye and float through outdoor and indoor air. Mold may begin growing indoors, when mold spores land on nutrient surfaces that are damp or wet. There are over four thousand types of mold and none of them will grow without water, moisture or elevated levels of humidity.

Spores may or may not germinate immediately, since they are built for survival. The spores may lie dormant, waiting for the right conditions for growth. Those conditions include a nutrient source (food), ideal temperature and a source of moisture. Favourable conditions for mold to grow:

Nutrient source–Molds feed on organic materials in a structure, such as wood, paper, drywall, insulation and natural fibres. We should be very conscious in observing nutrient sources of mold around us.

Ideal Temperature–Molds generally grows best in common building temperatures between 68 and 86 F. (Some molds, however, grow in cold temperatures, even down to 32 F, while others thrive in temperatures over 100 F). Generally too much of heat does not create conductive environment for mold to grow.

Moisture Source–Most molds can survive in relative humidity levels as low as 65%. To prevent most mold growth, indoor relative humidity should be maintained between 30% and 50%, and source of moisture such as plumbing or structural leaks should be resolved immediately.

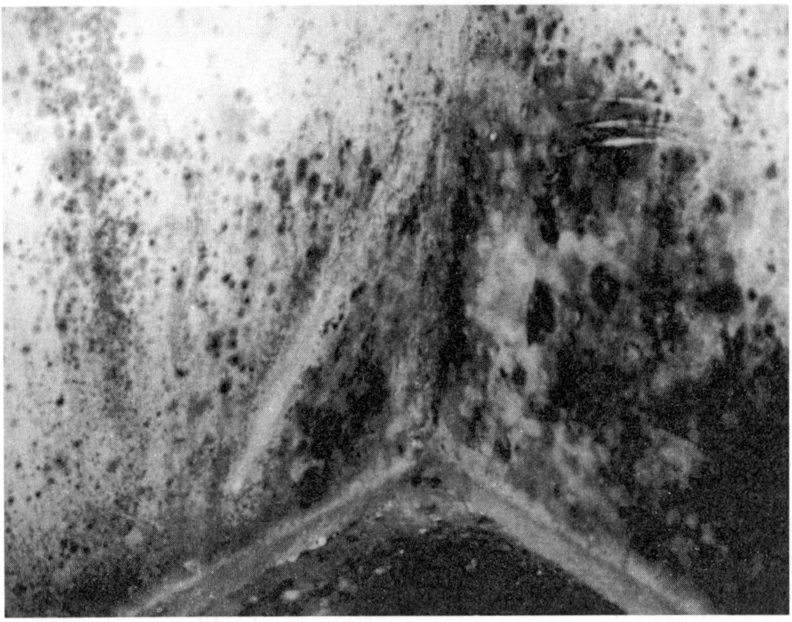

Mold in Walls

Molds can germinate where these conditions are present. How fast growth occurs depends on the combination of conditions. Houses offer an ample food supply such as, drywall, carpet and padding, wood, insulation and paper. When these materials become damp or wet, settled mold spores can begin colonizing and growing.

Molds are fungi that grow in the form of multicellular filaments called hyphae. Microscopic fungi that grow as single cells are called yeasts. A connected network of these tubular branching hyphae has multiple, genetically identical nuclei and is considered a single organism, referred to as a colony or in more technical terms a mycelium.

Like all fungi, molds derive energy not through photosynthesis but from the organic matter in which they live. Molds reproduce through small spores, which may contain a single nucleus or be multinucleate. Mold spores can be asexual or sexual; many species can produce both types. Mold spores may remain airborne indefinitely, may cling to clothing or fur, or may be able to survive extremes of temperature and pressure. Being airborne mold clings on to the clothes and moves from place to place. It can make a close proximity and becomes more dangerous for the health of the occupants.

Although molds grow on dead organic matter everywhere in nature, their presence is only visible to the unaided eye when mold colonies grow. A mold colony does not comprise discrete organisms, but an interconnected network of hyphae called a mycelium. Nutrients and in some cases organelles may be transported throughout the mycelium. In artificial environments like buildings, humidity and temperature are often stable enough to foster the growth of mold colonies, commonly seen as a downy or furry coating growing on food or other surfaces.

Many molds can begin growing at 4 °C (39 °F), the temperature within a typical refrigerator, or less. When conditions do not enable growth, molds may remain alive in a dormant state depending on the species, within a large range of temperatures before they die. The many different mold species vary enormously in their tolerance to temperature and humidity extremes. Xerophilic molds use the humidity in the air as their only water source; other molds need more moisture. Mold has a musty odor.

Common Molds

- Acremonium
- Aspergillus
- Cladosporium
- Fusarium
- Mucor
- Penicillium
- Rhizopus
- Stachybotrys
- Trichoderma

Health Effects

If mold spores are present in large quantities, they can present a health hazard to humans, potentially causing allergic reactions and respiratory problems.

Some molds can also produce mycotoxins that can pose serious health risks to humans and animals. It has been claimed that exposure to high levels of mycotoxins can lead to neurological problems and in some cases death specifically in case of prolonged exposure. The term "toxic mold" refers to molds that produce mycotoxins, such as Stachybotrys chartarum.

Mold in the home can usually be found in damp, dark or steam filled areas e.g. bathroom or kitchen, cluttered storage areas, recently flooded areas, basement areas, plumbing spaces, areas with poor ventilation and outdoors in humid environments. Mostly it is seen that bathrooms and basement create a perfect environment for molds to grow. Basements have less sunlight therefore more cold, more damp and dark as well.

Symptoms caused by mold allergy are watery, itchy eyes, a chronic cough, headaches or migraines, difficulty breathing, rashes, tiredness, sinus problems, nasal blockage and frequent sneezing.

Growth in Buildings and Homes

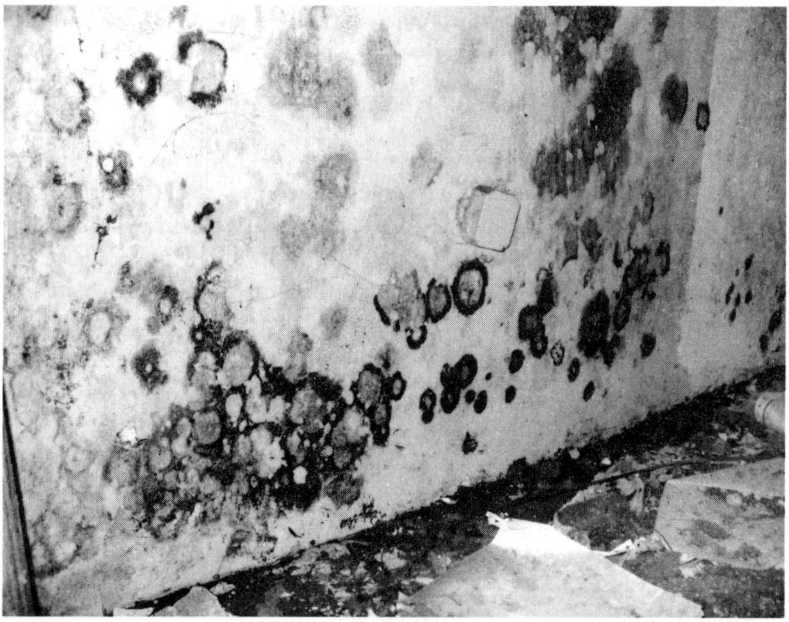

Mold in Old Buildings

Mold growth in buildings can lead to a variety of health issues. Various practices can be followed to mitigate mold issues in buildings, the most important of which is to reduce moisture levels that can facilitate mold growth. Removal of affected materials after the source of moisture has been reduced or eliminated may be necessary for remediation. Some of the health effects are:

Mold-associated conditions

Health problems associated with high levels of airborne mold spores include:

- Allergic reactions,
- Fungal infection,
- Digestive tract infections,
- Lung and skin infections,
- Rhinorrhea (runny nose),
- Watery eyes,
- Respiratory problems,
- Coughing,
- Asthma attacks,
- Irritations of the eye, nose and throat,
- Hypersensitivity, and
- Sinus congestion.

Solutions to the Problems of Mold:

- Plant trees and keep highly oxygenated air
- Install and use exhaust fans that are vented to the outdoors in kitchens and bathrooms and vent clothes dryers' outdoors.
- Keeping humidity levels in these areas below 50 percent can prevent water condensation on building materials.
- Thoroughly clean and dry water-damaged carpets and building materials (within 24 hours if possible) or consider removal and replacement.
- Keep the house clean. House dust mites, pollens, animal dander, and other allergy-causing agents can be reduced, although not eliminated, through regular cleaning.
- Take steps to minimize biological pollutants in basements.

Radon (Rn)

The most common source of indoor radon is uranium in the soil or rocks emitting uranium on which homes are built. As uranium naturally breaks down, it releases radon gas, which is a colorless, odorless, radioactive gas. Radon is a heavy gas. Radon gas enters homes through dirt floors, cracks in concrete walls and floors, floor drains, and sumps. When radon becomes trapped in buildings and concentrations build up indoors, exposure to radon becomes a concern.

Any home may have a radon problem. This means new and old homes, well-sealed and drafty homes, and homes with or without basements, however, it is only considered a significant risk in some areas. Sometimes radon enters the home through well water. In a small number of homes, the building materials can give off radon, too. However, building materials rarely cause radon problems by themselves.

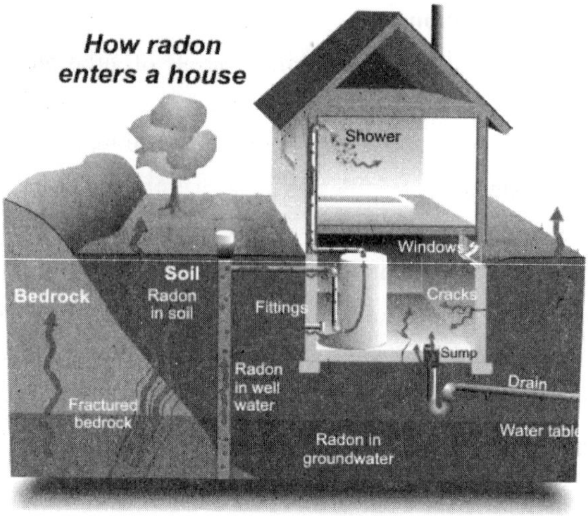

Radon Emission

Health Effects of Radon

The predominant health effect associated with exposure to elevated levels of radon is **lung cancer**. Some of the research suggests that swallowing water with high radon levels may pose risks, too, although these are believed to be much lower than those from breathing air containing radon. Major health organizations (like the Centres for Disease Control and Prevention, the American Lung Association (ALA), and the American Medical Association) agree with estimates that radon causes thousands of preventable lung cancer deaths each year. EPA estimates that radon causes about 14,000 deaths per year in the United States—however, this number could range from 7,000 to 30,000 deaths per year. If you smoke and your home has high radon levels, your risk of lung cancer is especially high.

Solutions to the problems of Radon:

Radon Reduction Techniques–There are several methods that a contractor can use to lower radon levels in your home. Some techniques prevent radon from entering your home while others reduce radon levels after it has entered. Environment Protection Agency normally recommends methods which prevent the entry of radon. Soil suction, for example, prevents radon from entering your home by drawing the radon from below the house and venting it through a pipe, or pipes, to the air above the house where it is quickly diluted.

Environmental Tobacco Smoke (ETS)

Environmental tobacco smoke (ETS) is the mixture of smoke that comes from the burning end of a cigarette, pipe, or cigar, and smoke exhaled by the smoker. It is a complex mixture of over 4,000 compounds, more than 40 of which are known to cause cancer in humans or animals and many of which are strong irritants. ETS is often referred to as "secondhand smoke" and exposure to ETS is generally called smoking."

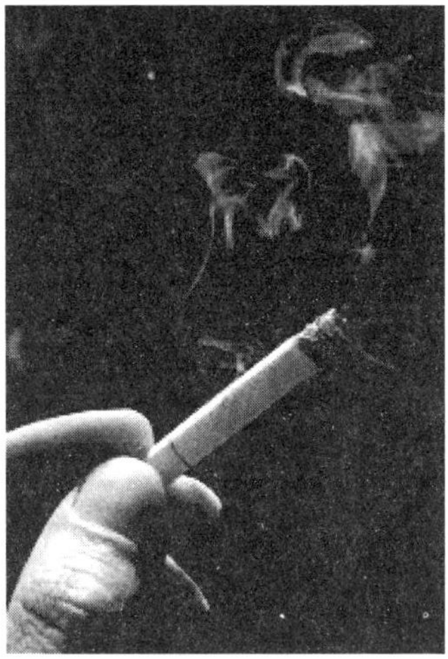

Tobacco Smoke

Health Effects of Environmental Tobacco Smoke

The Indian government has alarmed people of effects of Passive Smoking. It clearly instructs to place a warning on every packet of cigarette. The Delhi government does not allow smoking in public places and people are punished if they do so. People are asked to pay penalty if they smoke in public areas. The researches highlight that exposure to ETS can lead to lung cancer deaths.

Infants and young children whose parents smoke in their presence are at increased risk of lower respiratory tract infections (pneumonia and bronchitis) and are more likely to have symptoms of respiratory irritation like cough, excess phlegm, and wheeze. EPA estimates that passive smoking annually causes between 1,50,000 and 3,00,000 lower respiratory tract infections in infants and children under 18 months of age resulting in between 7,500 and 15,000 hospitalizations each year. These children may also have a build-up of fluid in the middle ear which can lead to ear infections. Older children who have been exposed to second hand smoke may have slightly reduced lung function.

Asthmatic children are especially at risk. EPA estimates that between 2,00,000 and 10,00,000 asthmatic children have their condition made worse by exposure to second hand smoke each year. Exposure to second hand smoke causes eye, nose, and throat irritation. It may affect the cardiovascular system and some studies have linked exposure to second hand smoke with jjie onset of chest pain.

Solutions to the problems of ETS:

- Don't smoke at home or permit others to do so. Ask smokers to smoke outdoors.
- Using Activated Oxygen To Remove Smoke Odours and ETS Contaminants
- If smoking indoors cannot be avoided, increase ventilation in the area where smoking takes place.

- Open windows or use exhaust fans.
- Do not smoke if children are present, particularly infants and toddlers.

Contamination from Stoves, Fireplaces and Chimneys

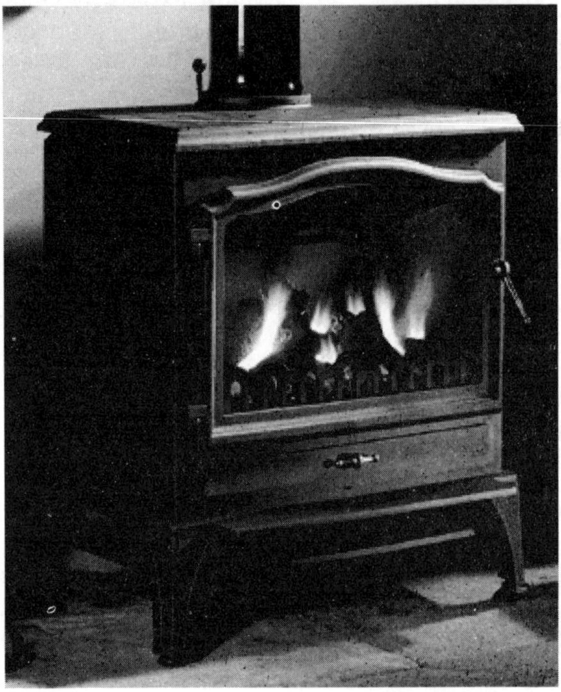

Fireplace

In addition to environmental tobacco smoke, other sources of combustion products are unvexnted, kerosene and gas space heaters, wood stoves, fireplaces, and gas stoves. The major pollutants are carbon monoxide, nitrogen dioxide and particles. Unvented kerosene heaters may also generate acid aerosols. Combustion gases and particles also come from chimneys that are not improperly installed or maintained. Pollutants from fireplaces and stoves with no dedicated outdoor air supply can be "back-drafted" in the home.

Health Effects of Combustion Products

Carbon monoxide (CO) is a colourless, odourless gas that interferes with the delivery of oxygen throughout the body. At high level of concentrations it can cause **unconsciousness** and **death**. Lower concentrations can also cause a range of symptoms **from headaches, dizziness, weakness, nausea and disorientation to fatigue** in healthy people. The symptoms of carbon-monoxide poisoning are sometimes confused with food poisoning. Foetuses, infants, elderly people, and people with anaemia or with a "history of heart or respiratory disease can be especially sensitive to carbon monoxide exposures.

Nitrogen dioxide (NO_2) is a colourless, odourless gas that irritates the mucous membranes in the eye, nose and throat and causes shortness of breath after exposure to high concentrations. It is seen that high concentrations or continued exposure to low levels of nitrogen dioxide increases the risk of respiratory infection. People at particular risk from exposure to nitrogen dioxide include children and individuals with asthma and other respiratory diseases.

Particles are released when fuels are incompletely burned and can irritate or damage lung issue. A number of pollutants, including radon and benzo(a) pyrene, both of which can cause cancer, attach to small particles that are inhaled and then carried deep into the lung.

Solutions:

➢ Reducing Exposure to Combustion Products in Homes

➢ Take special precautions when operating fuel burning unvented space heaters.

➢ Install and use exhaust fans or chimney over gas cooking stoves.

➢ Keep wood stove emissions to a minimum.

➢ Have central air handling systems, including furnaces, flues, and chimneys, inspected annually and promptly repair cracks or damaged parts.

➢ Blocked, leaking, or damaged chimneys or flues release harmful combustion gases and particles and even fatal concentrations of carbon monoxide. Strictly follow all service and maintenance procedures recommended by the manufacturer, including those that tell you how frequently to change the filter.

Contamination from Household Products

Paints, varnishes, and wax contain organic solvents. All of these products can release organic compounds while using. It has been found that a about a dozen common organic pollutants to be 2 to 5 times higher inside homes than outside, regardless of whether the homes were located in rural or highly industrial areas.

Health Effects of Household Chemicals

The ability of organic chemicals to cause health effects varies greatly, from those that are highly toxic, to those with no known health effect. As with other pollutants, the extent and nature of the health effect will depend on many factors including level of exposure and length of time exposed.

Eye and respiratory tract irritation, headaches, dizziness, visual disorders, and memory impairment are among the immediate symptoms that some people have experienced soon after exposure to some organics. Many organic compounds are known to cause cancer in animals and some are suspected of causing cancer in humans as well.

Solutions:

- Reducing Exposure to Household Chemicals
- Follow label instructions carefully- Potentially hazardous products often have warnings aimed at reducing exposure of the user.
- Buy limited quantities- If you use products only occasionally or seasonally, such as paints, paint strippers, and kerosene for space heaters buy only as much as you will use right away.
- Keep exposure to emissions from products containing methylene chloride to a minimum.
- Keep exposure to benzene to a minimum- Benzene is a known human carcinogen. The main indoor sources of this chemical are environmental tobacco smoke, stored fuels and paint supplies, and automobile emissions in attached garages. Actions that will reduce benzene exposure include eliminating smoking within the home, providing for maximum ventilation during painting, and discarding paint supplies and special fuels that will not be used immediately.
- Keep exposure to perchloroethylene emissions from newly dry-cleaned materials to a minimum. Perchloroethylene is the chemical most widely used in dry cleaning. In laboratory studies, it has been shown to cause cancer in animals. Recent studies indicate that people breathe low levels of this chemical both in homes where dry-cleaned goods are stored and as they wear dry-cleaned clothing.

Formaldehyde

Formaldehyde is an important chemical used widely by industry to manufacture building materials and numerous household products. It is also a by-product of combustion and certain other natural processes. Therefore it may be present in high concentrations both in indoors and outdoors.

Sources of formaldehyde in the home include building materials, smoking, household products, and the use of unvented, fuel-burning appliances, like gas stoves or kerosene space heaters. Formaldehyde, by itself or in combination with other chemicals, serves a number of purposes in manufactured products. For example, it is used a component of glues and adhesives, and as a preservative in some paints and coating products.

In homes, the most significant sources of formaldehyde are likely to be pressed wood products made using adhesives that contain urea-formaldehyde (UF) resins. Pressed wood products made for indoor use include: particleboard (used as subflooring, shelving, cabinets and furniture); hardwood-plywood paneling (used for decorative wall covering and used in cabinets and furniture); and medium density fiberboard (used for drawer fronts, cabinets, and furniture tops). Medium density fiberboard contains a higher resin-to-wood ratio than any other UF pressed wood product and is generally recognized as being the highest formaldehyde emitting pressed wood product.

In the Vedic period, architects were very careful in selecting wood. They knew properties of each wood and used it to improve efficiency, comfort and relaxation of the occupants. They knew the associated problems as well and used utmost care in using building materials.

Now agencies permit the use of plywood and particleboard that conform to specified formaldehyde emission limit. The rate at which products release formaldehyde can also change with time. The emissions may decrease with products age. When the products are new, high indoor temperatures or humidity can cause increased release of formaldehyde from these products.

Health Effects of Formaldehyde

Formaldehyde, a colourless, pungent-smelling gas, can cause, watery eyes, burning sensations in the eyes and throat, nausea, and difficulty in breathing in some humans-exposed at elevated levels (above 0.1 parts per million). High concentrations may trigger attacks in people with asthma. There is an evidence that some people can develop a sensitivity to formaldehyde. It has also been shown to cause cancer in animals and may cause cancer in humans as well.

Solutions:

- Reducing Exposure to Formaldehyde in Homes
- Ask about the formaldehyde content of pressed wood products, including building materials, cabinetry, and furniture from manufacturers before you purchase them.
- Some studies suggest that coating pressed wood products with polyurethane may reduce formaldehyde emissions for some period of time. To be effective, any such coating must cover all surfaces and edges and remain intact.
- Increase the ventilation and carefully follow the manufacturer instructions while applying these coatings. (If you are sensitive to formaldehyde, check the label contents before purchasing coating products to avoid buying products that contain formaldehyde, as they will emit the chemical for a short time after application.)

- Maintain moderate temperature and humidity levels and provide adequate ventilation. The rate at which formaldehyde is released is accelerated by heat and may also depend somewhat on the humidity level. Therefore, the use of dehumidifiers and air conditioning to control humidity and to maintain a moderate temperature can help reduce formaldehyde emissions.

Pesticides

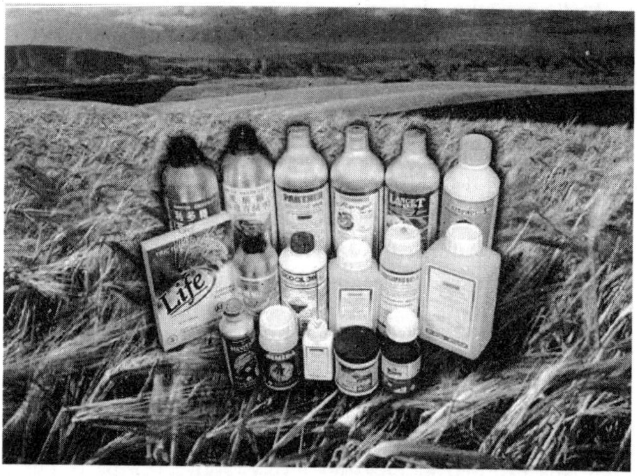

Pesticides can be contaminating

A study reveals that 80 percent of most people's exposure to pesticides occurs indoors. The possible sources include contaminated soil or dust floats or are tracked in from outside, stored pesticide containers. Pesticides used in and around the home include products to control insects (insecticides), termites (termiticides), rodents (rodenticides), fungi (fungicides), and microbes (disinfectants). They are sold as sprays, liquids, sticks, powders, crystals, balls, and foggers.

In 1990, the American Association of Poison Control Centers reported that some 79,000 children were involved in common household pesticide poisonings or exposures. In households with children under five years old, almost one-half stored at least one pesticide product within reach of children. Now days the indirect impact of pesticide residue in vegetables is also affecting human health.

EPA registers pesticides for use and requires manufacturers to put information on the label about when and how to use the pesticide. It is important to remember that the "cide" in pesticides means "to kill." These products can prove to be dangerous if not used properly.

Health Effects from Pesticides

Both the active and inert ingredients in pesticides can be organic compounds; therefore, both could add to the levels of airborne organics inside homes. Exposure to high levels of cyclodiene pesticides, commonly associated with misapplication, has various symptoms like headaches, dizziness, muscle twitching, weakness, tingling sensations, and nausea. In addition, EPA is concerned that cyclodienes might cause long-term damage to the liver and the central nervous system, as well as an increased risk of cancer.

Sale or commercial use of pesticides like chlordane, aldrin, dieldrin, and heptachlor has not been permitted. The only exception is the use of heptachlor by utility companies to control fire ants in underground cable boxes.

Solutions:

- Reducing Exposure to Pesticides in Homes
- Read the label and follow the directions. Use only the pesticides approved for use by the general public and then only in recommended amounts; increasing the amount does not offer more protection against pests and can be harmful to you and your plants and pets.
- Ventilate the area well after pesticide use. Mix or dilute pesticides outdoors or in a well-ventilated area and only in the amounts that will be immediately needed.
- If possible, take plants and pets outside when applying pesticides to them. Use non-chemical methods of pest control when possible. Since pesticides can be found far from the site of their original application, it is prudent to reduce the use of chemical pesticides outdoors as well as indoors.
- Dispose of unwanted pesticides safely.
- Keep exposure to moth repellents to a minimum. One pesticide often found in the home is paradichlorobenzene, a commonly used active ingredient in moth repellents. This chemical is known to cause cancer in animals, but substantial scientific uncertainty exists over the effects, if any, of long-term human exposure to paradichlorobenzene.
- Proper ventilation and basic household cleanliness will go a long way toward preventing unpleasant odours.

Lead

Lead has long been recognized as a harmful environmental pollutant, the Secretary of the Department of Health and Human Services called lead the "number one environmental threat to the health of children in the United States." There are many ways in which humans are exposed to lead: contaminated soil, deteriorating paint, and dust. Airborne lead enters the body when an individual breathes or swallows lead particles or dust once it has used. Before it was known how harmful lead could be, it was used in paint, gasoline, water pipes, and many other products.

Harmful exposures to lead can be created when lead-based paint is improperly removed from surfaces. High concentrations of airborne lead particles in homes also result from lead dust from outdoor sources, including contaminated soil tracked inside, and use o: lead in certain indoor activities such as soldering and stained-glass making.

Health Effects of Exposure to Lead

Lead affects practically all systems within the body. At high levels it can cause **convulsions, coma, and even death**. Lower levels of lead can adversely affect the **brain, central nervous system, blood cells, and kidneys**. The effects of lead exposure on fetuses and young children can be severe. They include delays in physical and mental development, lower IQ levels, shortened attention spans, and increased behavioral problems, rouses, intains, and children are more vulnerable to lead exposure than adults are since lead is more easily absorbed into growing bodies.

Solutions:

- Reduce the risk from lead-based paint. Most homes built before 1960 contain heavily leaded paint. Some homes built as recently as 1978 may also contain lead paint. This paint could be on window frames, walls, the outside of homes, or other surfaces. Do not burn painted wood since it may contain lead.
- Leave lead-based paint undisturbed if it is in good condition - do not sand or burn off paint that may contain lead. Lead paint in good condition is usually not a problem except in places where painted surfaces rub against each other and create dust (for example, opening a window).
- Do not remove lead paint yourself. Individuals have been poisoned by scraping or sanding lead paint because these activities generate large amounts of lead dust. Consult an expert.
- Do not bring lead dust into the home. If you work in construction, demolition, painting, with batteries, in a radiator repair shop or lead factory, or your hobby involves lead, you may unknowingly bring lead into your home on your hands or clothes. You may also be tracking in lead from soil inside. Soil very close to homes may be contaminated from lead paint on the outside of the building. Soil by roads and highways may be contaminated from years of exhaust fumes from cars and trucks that used leaded gas. Use doormats to wipe your feet before entering.

Preventive Measures for Home Owners

Moisture control is the key to mold control, so when water leaks or spills occur indoors - **ACT QUICKLY**. If wet or damp materials or areas are dried 24-48 hours after a leak or spill happens, in most cases mold will not grow.

- Clean and repair roof gutters regularly
- Make sure the ground slopes away from the building foundation, so that water does not enter or collect around the foundation.
- Keep air conditioning drip pans clean and the drain lines unobstructed and flowing properly.
- Keep indoor humidity low. If possible, keep indoor humidity below 60 percent (ideally between 30 and 50 percent) relative humidity. Relative humidity can be measured with a moisture or humidity meter, a small, inexpensive instrument available at many hardware stores.
- If you see condensation or moisture collecting on windows, walls or pipes ACT QUICKLY to dry the wet surface and reduce the moisture/water source. Condensation can be a sign of high humidity.

Actions that will help to reduce humidity:

- Vent appliances that produce moisture, such as clothes dryers, stoves, and kerosene heaters to the outside where possible. (Combustion appliances such as stoves and kerosene heaters produce water vapour and will increase the humidity unless vented to the outside.)
- Use air conditioners and/or de-humidifiers when needed.
- Run the bathroom fan or open the window when showering. Use exhaust fans or open windows whenever cooking, running the dishwasher or dish washing, etc.

Actions that will help prevent condensation:

- Reduce the humidity (see above).
- Increase ventilation or air movement by opening doors and/or windows, when practical. Use fans as needed.
- Cover cold surfaces, such as cold water pipes, with insulation.
- Increase air temperature.

Solutions to Poor Indoor Air Quality

This "Room-By-Room" checklist will give you helpful tips for maintaining healthy indoor air quality for you and your family. Each room listed will include various sources of indoor air contaminants as well as remedies and solutions to avoid IAQ problems in your home.

Kitchen	Possible remedies
Household Cleaners	Open window, and use according to manufacturer's directions
Moisture	(Cooking, Dishwasher Use or leaky pipes, sinks, etc. Install and use exhaust fan. Fix source of moisture.
Pressed-Wood Cabinets	When purchasing pressed-wood cabinetry or furniture, ask about formaldehyde content and release. Some types of pressed-wood products, such as those with phenol resin, emit less formaldehyde. Also, pressed-wood products coated with polyurethane or laminates may reduce formaldehyde emissions. After installation, open windows. Maintain moderate temperature and humidity.
Unvented Gas Stove or Range	Keep burners properly adjusted *(blue flame tip, not yellow)* Install and use exhaust fan. Never use a gas stove to heat your home.
Bathroom	**Possible remedies**
Air Freshener	Open window or use exhaust fan instead. If using air fresheners, follow manufacturer's directions.
Moisture, Mold and Mildew	Install and use exhaust fan. Fix plumbing leaks promptly
Personal Care Products:	e.g. hair spray, nail polish, etc.) Open window or use exhaust fan. Follow manufacturer's directions. Use non-aerosol products.
Bedroom	**Possible remedies**
Dry Cleaned Goods	Do not accept dry cleaned goods with chemical odor until they have been properly dried. Try a different dry cleaner.
Humidifier	Clean according to manufacturer's directions. Refill with clean water daily. Keep moderate temperature and humidity levels.
Moth Repellents *(with paradichlorobenzene)*	Avoid breathing vapors. Place moth repellents in trunks or other containers and store separately (attic, storage closet, etc.), away from living areas.
Living Room	**Possible remedies**

Paneling, Pressed-Wood Furniture	(See Kitchen – Pressed-wood cabinets)
All Rooms	**Possible remedies**
Moisture	Use exhaust fans. Use dehumidifier if necessary. Fix leaky pipes or source of moisture.
Carpets	Clean and dry or remove water-damaged carpets promptly. If installing new carpet, ask your retailer to air out the carpet before installation. Ask for low-emitting adhesives, if adhesives are needed.
Draperies	(New draperies may be treated with a formaldehyde-based finish and may emit formaldehyde for a short time. Open doors and windows. Maintain moderate temperatures and humidity.
Environmental Tobacco Smoke (ETS)	Do not smoke in your home or permit others to do so (especially near children). If smoking cannot be avoided, open windows or use exhaust fans.
Floor Tiles Containing Asbestos	Periodically inspect for damage or deterioration. Do not cut, rip, sand or remove any asbestos-containing materials. If you plan to make changes that might disturb the asbestos or if materials are more than slightly damaged, repair or removal by a professional is recommended.
House Dust Mites	Clean house and vacuum regularly. Wash bedding in hot water.
Lead-Based Paint	(if manufactured before 1978) Leave lead based paint undisturbed if it is in good condition. Do not sand, burn off or remove. Hire a professional with special training for correcting lead paint problems.
Animals	(dander, hair, feathers or shedding skin) Clean house and animal facilities regularly
Garage	**Possible remedies**
Car Exhaust	Do not idle car in garage. To keep exhaust out of house, use weather stripping on door from garage to house.

Paint Supplies	Open windows when using. Follow manufacturer's directions. Buy limited quantities. If products contain methylene cloride (e.g. paint strippers), use outdoors. Reseal containers well. Clean brushes and other materials outside.
Pesticides	(products that kill household pests) Use non-chemical methods of pest control where possible. Follow manufacturer's directions. Mix or dilute outdoors. Open windows when using indoors. Take plants or pets outside when applying pesticides. Do not store pesticides inside house.
Stored Fuels	(e.g. gasoline, kerosene, etc.) Buy limited quantities. Use well-sealed containers. Do not store inside home.
Basement or Ground Floor	**Possible remedies**
Asbestos Pipe Wrap and Furnace Insulation	See All Rooms: Floor Tiles containing asbestos.
Dehumidifier	Empty and clean water tray often.
Ground Moisture	Clean and disinfect basement floor drain regularly. Keep basement dry and free of moisture and mildew.
Radon	Test your home for radon. Do-it-yourself kits are easy and inexpensive. Fix your home if radon level is 4 picocuries per liter (pCi/L) or higher. For more information, contact your state radon office or call 1-800-SOS-RADON.
Stored Hobby Products	(e.g. paint, glue, epoxy, etc.) Follow manufacturer's directions. Use outdoors, if possible. Indoors, open windows or use exhaust fan. Reseal containers well. Clean brushes and other materials outside.
Heating and Cooling Systems	**Possible remedies**
Air Conditioner	Empty and clean water tray often. Follow all service and maintenance procedures, including changing filters and cleaning evaporator coils.

Furnace	Have your heating system inspected and serviced every year. Repair fuel or gas leaks promptly. Follow service and maintenance guidance, including changing filter.
Fireplace	Open flue when fireplace is in use. Have flue and chimney inspected annually for blocks, leaks or other damages.
Gas Space Heater	In room where heater is located, open a door to the rest of the house. Turn on exhaust fan and open a window slightly.
Wood Burning Stove	Vent to outside. Choose a properly sized wood stove that is certified to meet EPA emission standards. Make certain all wood stove doors fit tightly. Use aged or cured (dried) wood. Follow manufacturer's directions.

General Solution to Indoor Air Quality:

Removal of the pollutant source is the most effective way to solve an indoor air quality issue, when it can be done and when the cause is known. Regular maintenance of HVAC systems; replacing water-stained drywall, panels, wood, ceiling tiles and carpets is an important start to improving the quality of indoor air. A ban on tobacco use is a major plus. Venting emissions to the outdoors will also improve indoor air quality. If you're having remodelling done in the near future or even now it is always a good idea to leave the completed remodelling job unoccupied for a good period of time to allow gaseous pollutants to fade away over time.

Restrooms, copy machine and print rooms should always be ventilated to the outside whenever possible. Increasing ventilation and air distribution can be a cost effective way to reduce indoor air pollution. Routine maintenance of HVAC systems should always be a priority. Air filters should always be cleaned/replaced at regular intervals. Other contaminants such as paints, adhesives, solvents, and pesticides should be stored, and used, in well ventilated areas only.

Air purification and filtration is also helpful with source control and ventilation but can have limitations if the proper systems are not used. Standard air filters found in furnace and A/C air handlers are inexpensive but do not do a great job at filtering out small particles. A high performance replacement filter is always recommended, such as the 3M Filtrete, a filter we know to be superior in performance from our own testing. Mechanical filters do not remove gaseous pollutants such as volatile organic compounds.

Ozone can be effective to a certain extent, but it can also cause many health problems and is not considered a solution by any means. Ionic style air purifiers are near worthless when it comes to a major change in indoor air quality. In some cases they can actually make the interior dirtier since pollutants the ions attach themselves to can later begin sticking to walls, furniture, and everything else. Germicidal systems provide a very cost effective, and very dependable, solution to indoor air quality issues. Even better, the use of photocatalysis, combined with germicidal UV light is superior to all other forms mentioned above. This method is known as green chemistry. A non-toxic and completely dependable way to reduce indoor air pollutants, if not eliminate them.

By following the suggestions in the previous pages of this report and using the latest technology in air purification the problem of Sick Building Syndrome can be greatly reduced. Indoor air quality can be greatly improved, and this chain reaction effect can improve the health, and comfort, of the occupants.

Noise Pollution and Sick Building Syndrome

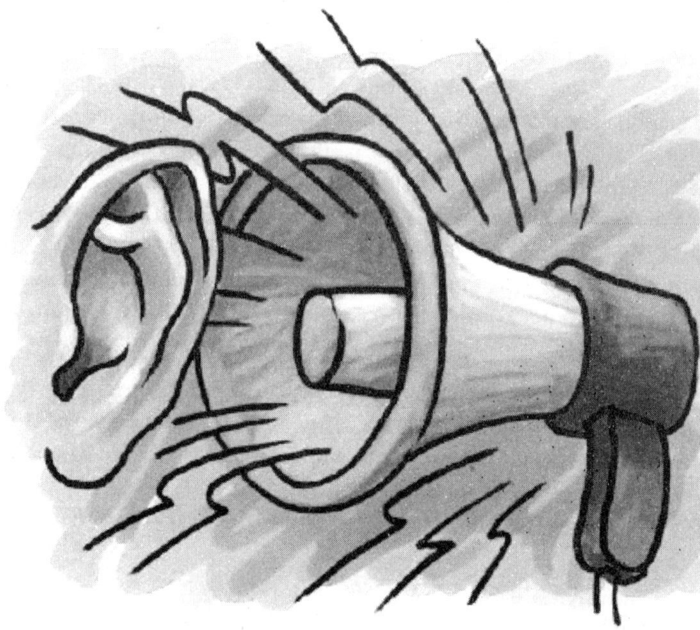

Noise Pollution

Pleasing Sounds are called music whereas unpleasing and unbearable sounds are referred to as noise. Noise beyond acceptable limits is termed as noise pollution. **Noise pollution** is displeasing human, animal or machine-created sound that disturbs the activity or balance of human or animal life.

Sources of Noise:

- Construction
- Transportation systems, including motor vehicle noise, aircraft noise and rail noise
- Industrial activities
- Indoor and outdoor noise pollution sources include car alarms
- Emergency service sirens
- Mechanical equipments
- Fireworks
- Compressed air horns
- Grounds-keeping equipment
- Barking dogs
- Appliances
- Audio entertainment systems
- Loud people
- Anti-Social Behaviour such as uses of Loudspeaker is a highly sensitive social issue in India

Too much of noise is banned

Health Effects on Human Health:

Noise health effects can be both mental and physical. The unwanted sounds can damage physiological and psychological health. Noise pollution can cause:

- Annoyance and aggression,
- Hypertension,
- High stress levels,
- Tinnitus,
- Hearing loss,
- Sleep disturbances, and other harmful effects.

Furthermore, stress and hypertension are the leading causes to health problems. Chronic exposure to noise may cause noise-induced hearing loss. Older males exposed to significant occupational noise demonstrate significantly reduced hearing sensitivity than their non-exposed peers, though differences in hearing sensitivity decrease with time. High noise levels can contribute to:

- Cardiovascular effects
- Rise in blood pressure of five to ten points
- An increase in stress
- And Vasoconstriction leading to the increased blood pressure, and
- Coronary Artery disease.

Over exposure to noise can have negative effect on animals and plants as well. It can lead to stress, increasing risk of death by changing the delicate balance in predator/prey detection and avoidance, and by interfering with their use of sounds in communication especially in relation to reproduction and in navigation. Acoustic overexposure can lead to temporary or permanent loss of hearing.

Detecting Noise Pollution

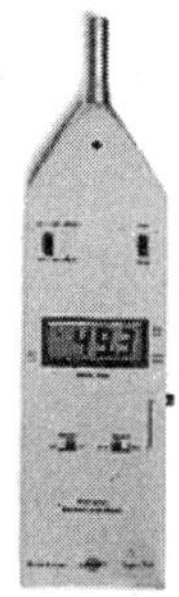

Sound Level Meter

Sound level meter is used to detect noise pollution in and around a building. Sound is measured in decibels. Ideally sound level inside a building should be less than 55 decibels. Noise pollution is rising in metropolitan cities. It may be less in early morning, afternoon and night. Generally it is at its peak during rush hours. There is no parallel in the world to the noise pollution generated during festivals and religious celebrations in India. For politicians the ability to make a big noise, by using huge loudspeakers at any opportunity, is a sign of strength. Festivals in India have become political battlegrounds as politicians try to score brownie points over one another by attempting to host the noisiest festival. The use of loudspeakers, permitted by the courts on certain occasions, often exceeds the permissible decibel limit, causing a great deal of stress and anxiety to the neighbourhoods.

Environmental Effects

Noise can have a detrimental effect on animals by causing stress, increasing risk of death by changing the delicate balance in predator/prey detection and avoidance, and by interfering with their use of sounds in communication especially in relation to reproduction and in navigation. Acoustic overexposure can lead to temporary or permanent loss of hearing.

An impact of noise on animal life is the reduction of usable habitat that noisy areas may cause, which in the case of endangered species may be part of the path to extinction. Noise pollution has caused the death of certain species of whales that beached themselves after being exposed to the loud sound of military sonar.

Noise also makes species communicate louder, which is called Lombard vocal response. Scientists and researchers have conducted experiments that show whales' song length is longer when submarine-detectors are on. If creatures do not "speak" loud enough, their voice will be masked by anthropogenic sounds. These unheard voices might be warnings, finding of prey, or preparations of net-bubbling. When one species begins speaking louder, it will mask other species' voice, causing the whole ecosystem to eventually speak louder.

Zebra finches become less faithful to their partners when exposed to traffic noise. This could alter a population's evolutionary trajectory by selecting traits, sapping resources normally devoted to other activities and thus lead to profound genetic and evolutionary consequences.

Solutions to Noise Pollution:

There are a variety of strategies for mitigating roadway noise including:

- Use of noise barriers,
- Limitation of vehicle speeds,
- Alteration of roadway surface texture,
- Limitation of heavy vehicles, and
- Use of traffic controls that smooth vehicle flow to reduce braking and acceleration, and tire design.

Other solutions to control noise pollution in a building are:

Tree Plantation: Effective solution for noise pollution is to plant bushes and trees around the sound generating sources. Sound passage is blocked by the dense shrubs and trees. Trees can be planted in the surrounding area to live peacefully.

Soundproof Homes: To block unwanted noise from outside soundproof doors and windows can be installed. If you stay in crowded city area these soundproof options are important for complete relaxation.

Plastered Walls: Textured walls also absorb a lot of noise. It should be used to cut noise levels coming from outside.

Foam, Thermocol & Cloth: Insulative materials like foam, thermocol or thick cloth can help in reducing noise levels to a considerable level.

Loudspeaker Prohibition: The major cause of noise pollution in public areas is loudspeaker. For the welfare of the people it should be banned at any cost. Those who violate and play loudspeakers in crowded areas and public places strict laws should be imposed against them.

Factory Location: From the residential areas factories and industries should be located in far off places. Installation of sound detectors will help in analysing the sound frequencies on a regular basis.

To wear ear protection while working in noisy conditions is an effective way to manage noise.

Sound insulation at the top of the roof can reduce the aircraft noise. Add a layer of plasterboard or wood to the dividing wall to protect yourself from the noise from neighbours.

4

Diagnoses and Solutions of Sick Building Syndrome

Tools, Devices and Instruments

Introduction to Scientific Instruments

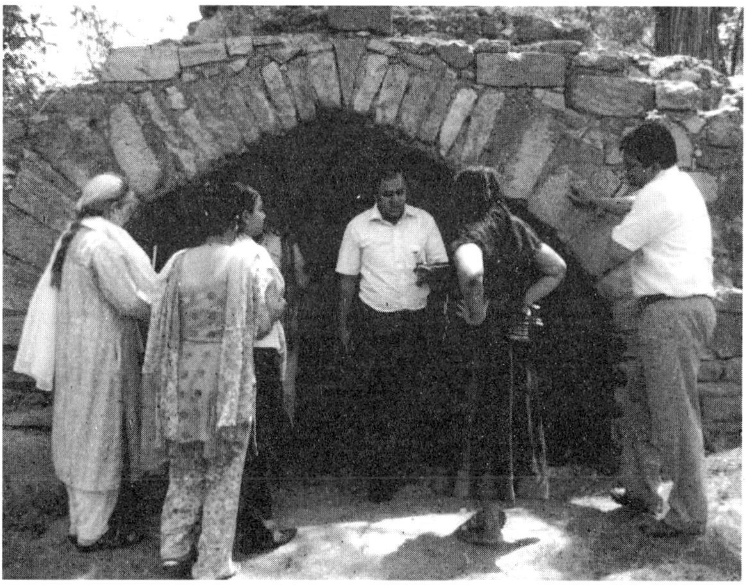

There are various scientific instrument used now a days. A small description about some of them is given below:

Lecher Antenna

Ernst Lecher discovered the principle of measuring energy in 1890. The Lecher Antenna was developed by a group of German physicists in 1975 based on Dr. Lecher's principle. In ancient days "Intuition" was the only the way to find the body vibration. It could not be proven. But now there is an instrument that measures the energy fields in the environmental, architectural, bioenvironmental and around the physical body.

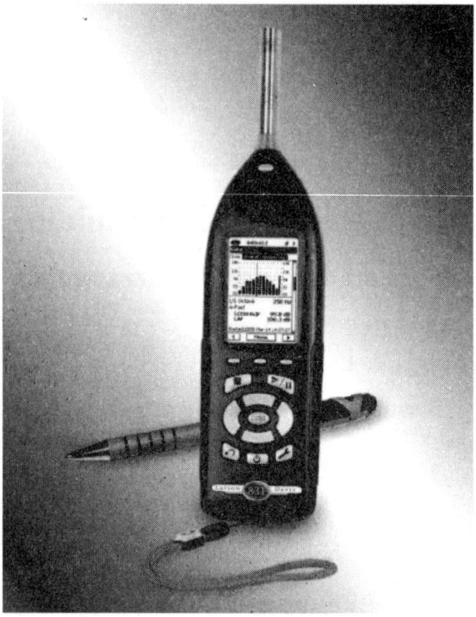

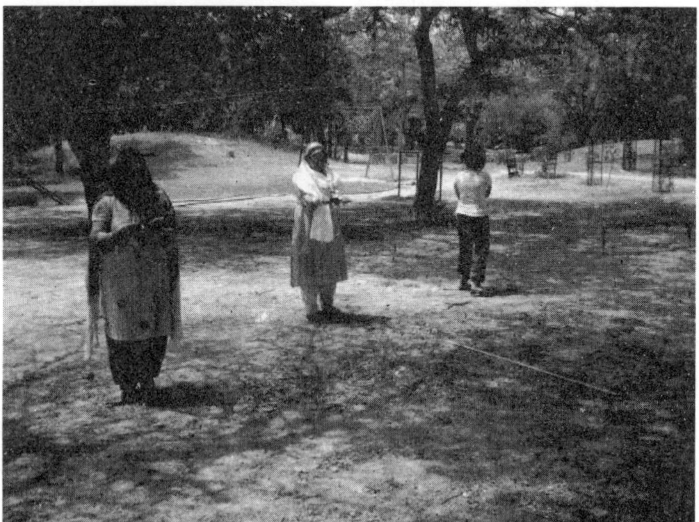

Lecher Antenna–Scientific Background

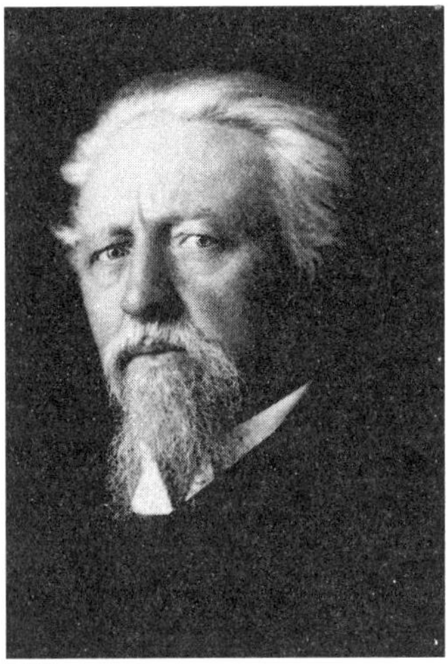

German Physicist–Ernst Lecher

Quantum physics emphasizes that at the sub-atomic level matter is energy and consists of energetic systems interacting with each other. At this sub-atomic level, all matter emits subtle energy or 'photon' particles of light. The Lecher antenna is able to tune into and measure these subtle energy emissions, the wavelengths of which are extremely small. The units of measurement are known as nanometres, which represent wave lengths of one meter divided by one billion.

In his famous formula $e=mc^2$. Einstein showed that energy and matter are one and the same substance. This universal substance is a sea of energy, of which we are all composed. The same subtle life force that animates us also animates elements of our lives such as our food, the supplements we take and the music we listen to. The antenna is able to tune into individual frequencies in this mass ocean of energy and relate them to the human organism by determining which wavelengths are beneficial to the human organism.

The Lecher antenna works on the resonance principle in that the body has energy reserves which are used to maintain balance in the body's energy systems. These reserves are used up if the body is continually attacked from external (electromagnetic stress, geopathic stress) and internal (devitalized food) sources. If these energy reserves are not replenished this creates missing links. A substance placed within the human energy field that fills this void evokes a resonance, which the antenna can identify.

Lecher Antenna is a tool that can measure the defective human energy meridians and shift in the fields and tell us which part of the house need correction. The base, earth, is from where we receive geopathic bliss, and the earth energy imbalance is the major cause of most human illnesses. By using Lecher Antenna effectively, one can diagnose various defects.

For the Sick Building correction we need to consider the impact of Environmental aggression on three major human energy centres:

- *The reading 12 lambda at Lecher Level: the Cosmic Energy*
- *The reading 15.3 lambda at the Lecher level: the Global Energy*
- *The reading at 8 lambda at the Lecher level: the Telluric Energy*

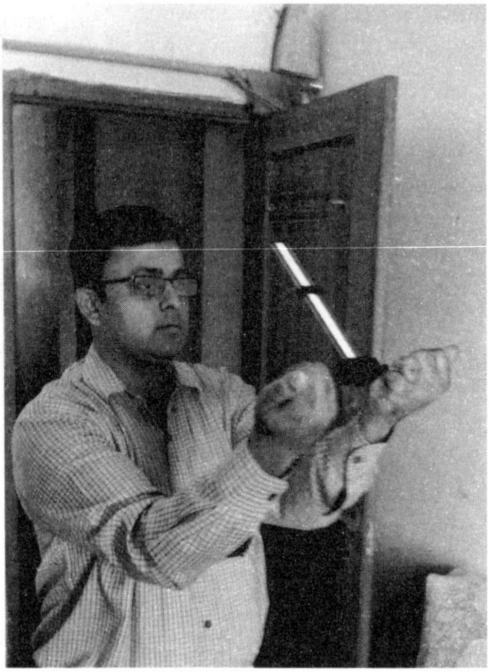

Energy Diagnosis through Lecher Antenna

The Lecher antenna is able to detect the earth's energy grid, ley lines, hartmann grid and curry lines. It can measure geopathic stress, radon emission and positive and negative energy, healthy vegetation and positive surroundings. Lecher antenna is the first instrument in the field of energy science that can measure various types of phenomenal energies. The antenna also allows one to read and verify vibrations of the human body.

The Lecher antenna functions on the principle of resonance. It determines energy impulses based on the principle that anything that vibrates faster will have a shorter wavelength. The length of the antenna rods is selected on the basis of half-wavelengths or their multiples.

EMF/ Radiation Tester

To measure and analyse the EMF radiations, one should be equipped with an instrument which can detect the correct vibration & provides the appropriate Ambient Electro Magnetic Pollution. EMF Radiation Tester is an indicator of electric and electromagnetic ambient pollution. It digitally shows the intensity of EMF.

EMF / Radiation Tester also detect various sources of pathogenic emissions, such as:

- Electric pollution emitted by electric wires, conduction equipment, wired walls, wall painting, wall paper and partitions, etc.
- High tension electric cables and the distance of the pollution from the cables.
- Emissions from instruments and equipment even if battery driven or charged.
- Emissions from television and computer.

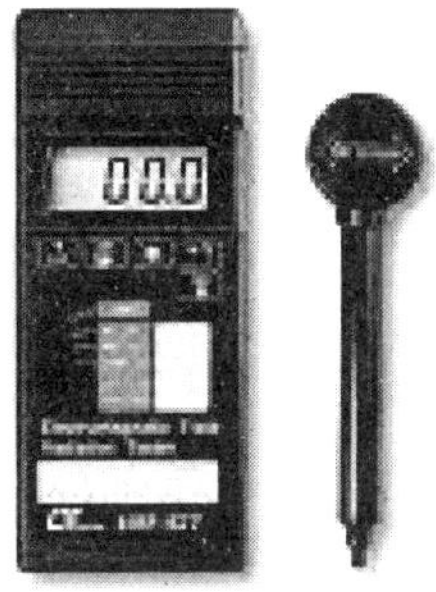

EM Radiation Tester

EMF Radiation Tester is a digital instrument which shows the exact reading with varying intensities. A standard 9 volt battery is used to operate this very low energy consuming instrument using high tech electronic component.

Magnetic Compass

The device to measure the magnetic axis and detect the true cardinal north is a magnetic compass. The best way to establish directions accurately is through magnetic compass. Three types of magnetic compass are used for this purpose:

i. Pivotal needle

ii. Floating disc

iii. Digital compass

Pivotal needle is an ordinary compass commonly used in school laboratory with a coloured tip, usually in red. Due to the magnetic field of the earth, this needle invariably points towards North. The needle of the compass when placed on a levelled surface starts oscillating. When the needle stops, one should align the coloured tip with the N mark on the compass. This N shows the exact North.

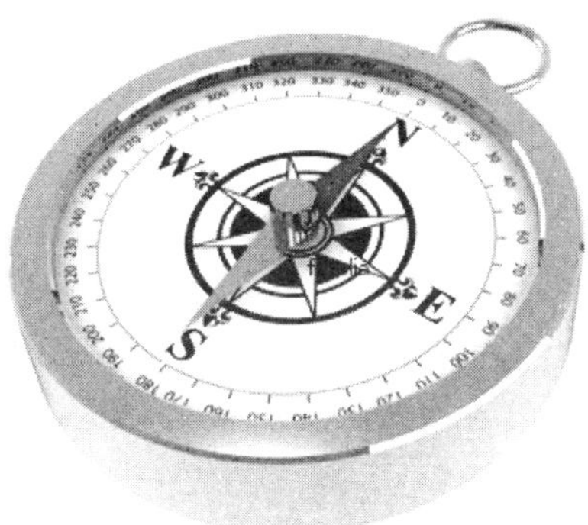

Magnetic Compass

Floating Disc is an improved version of the pivotal needle. It is an automatic device that points towards the direction automatically. In this kind of compass, a disc mounted on the needle due to which there is no need to align the tip, as is the case with Pivotal needle. This kind of compass being of superior quality, makes it easier to find the accurate directions without being much influenced by external sources .

Digital compass is a new development in the field of Vastu science. It shows digital reading of direction

Sound Level Meter

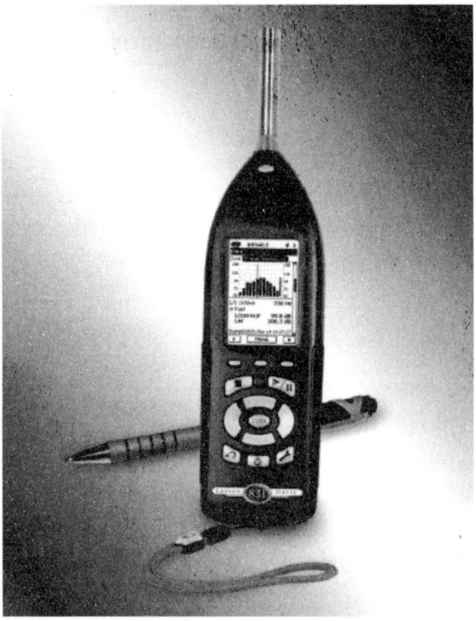

Sound Level Meter

It is a device for measuring the intensity of noise, music, and other sounds. A typical meter consists of a microphone for picking up the sound and converting it into an electrical signal, followed by electronic circuitry for operating on this signal so that the desired characteristics can be measured. The indicating device is usually a meter calibrated to read the sound level in decibels (dB; a logarithmic unit used to measure the sound intensity).

The ideal level of sound for human habitat is between 50 to 70 decibels. If the sound level goes beyond 120 decibels, it may cause problems.

Lux Meter

Lux meter is a device used to measure the amount of light. It helps in detecting the adequate levels of light needed for healthy living. Different light levels are recommended for different areas and functionalities.

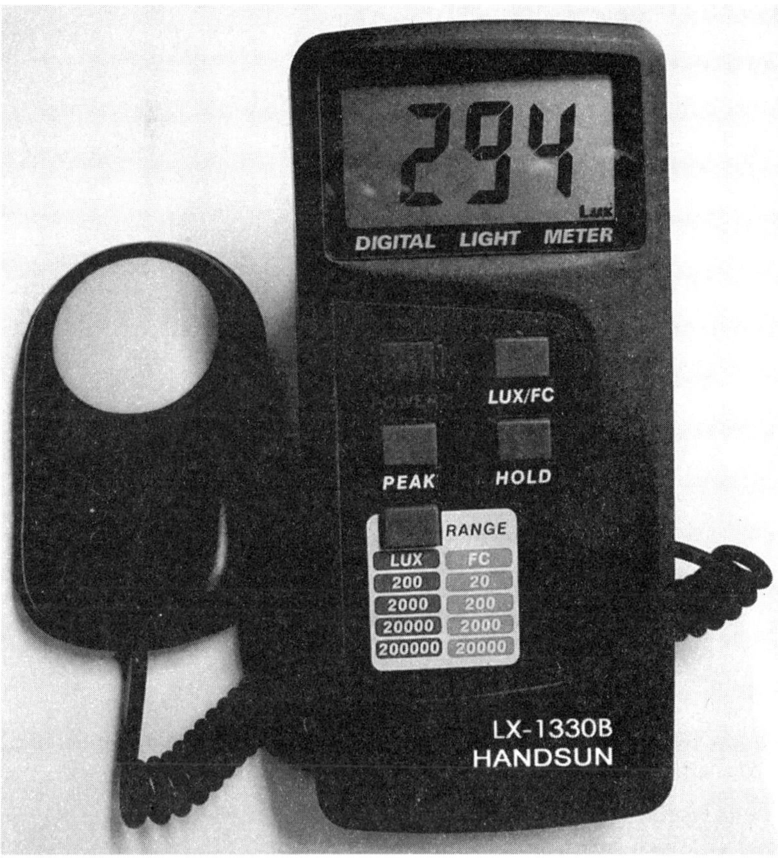

Lux Meter

A Light meter is also used in the fields of cinematography and scenic design, in order to determine the optimum light level for a scene. They are used in the general field of lighting, where they can help to reduce the amount of waste light used in the home, light pollution outdoors, and plant growing to ensure proper light levels.

Wind Vane and Anemometer

An **anemometer** is a device for measuring wind speed. The term is derived from the Greek word *anemos*, meaning wind. The first known description of an anemometer was given by Leon Battista Alberti around 1450. Anemometers can be divided into two classes: those that measure the wind's speed, and those that measure the wind's pressure; but as there is a close connection between the pressure and the speed, an anemometer designed for one will give information about both. Anemometer helps in the detecting the air movement and ventilation levels of a building.

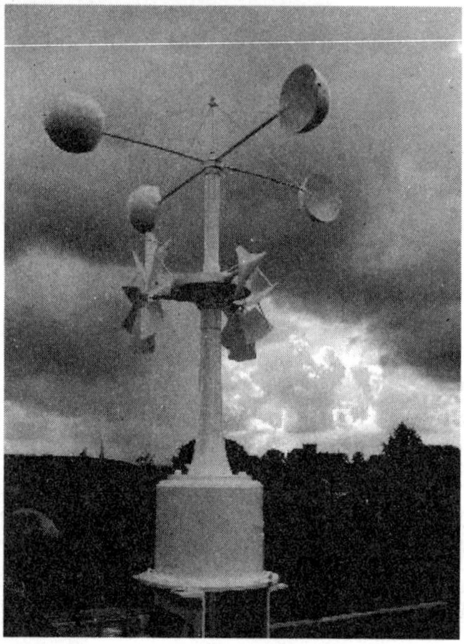

Wind Vane

Tips for creating a Healthy Building

A healthy dwelling must ensure some of the below mentioned characteristics:

- A healthy location helps in creation of healthy environment.
- A healthy dwelling must have a perfect balance between internal and external environment.
- The building should be free from all syndromes like SAD and SIDS.
- The interiors should not suffer from multiple chemical sensitivity and environmental aggression.
- The building should be full of natural sunlight at desirable timings.
- Perfect balance of temperature, sound, wind velocity, wind direction and relative humidity.
- The indoor air quality should be good. It should be free from inorganic contaminations like carbon monoxide and nitrogen dioxide etc. It should

also be free from germs, bacteria and fungi beyond maximum limits permitted.

- There should be a flow of fresh air inside, ventilation rate should be high.
- There should be substantial amount of negative ions in the indoor environment.
- Green plants and trees located in or around the plot make it a healthy dwelling.
- The orientation and openings of the building should be planned considering the pattern of solar movement.
- The form of the building should be designed considering the environmental forces and pressures.
- A perfect bioclimate should be built inside.
- The circulation of air, energy, bio-matter and water should be complete.
- Eco-friendly or natural materials should be used.
- The material, shape, angle and look of furniture should follow basic health guidelines.
- Safety and health measures should be completely adhered as per the by-laws of the government.
- Prefer constructing a GREEN BUILDING as per the guidelines of GRIHA and IGBC.
- Prefer constructing a Vastu friendly building.

5
Indian and International Guidelines on Sick Building Syndrome

Guidelines by Unites States Environmental Protection Agency

Introduction

The term "Sick Building Syndrome" (SBS) is used to describe situations in which building occupants experience acute health and comfort effects that appear to be linked to time spent in a building, but no specific illness or cause can be identified. The complaints may be localized in a particular room or zone, or may be widespread throughout the building. In contrast, the term "building related illness" (BRI) is used when symptoms of diagnosable illness are identified and can be attributed directly to airborne building contaminants.

A 1984 World Health Organization Committee report suggested that up to 30 percent of new and remodelled buildings worldwide may be the subject of excessive complaints related to indoor air quality (IAQ). Often this condition is temporary, but some buildings have long-term problems. Frequently, problems result when a building is operated or maintained in a manner that is inconsistent with its original design or prescribed operating procedures. Sometimes indoor air problems are a result of poor building design or occupant activities.

Indicators of SBS include:

- Building occupants complain of symptoms associated with acute discomfort, e.g., headache; eye, nose, or throat irritation; dry cough; dry or itchy skin; dizziness and nausea; difficulty in concentrating; fatigue; and sensitivity to odours.
- The cause of the symptoms is not known.
- Most of the complainants report relief soon after leaving the building.

Indicators of BRI include:

- Building occupants complain of symptoms such as cough; chest tightness; fever, chills; and muscle aches.
- The symptoms can be clinically defined and have clearly identifiable causes.

- Complainants may require prolonged recovery times after leaving the building.

It is important to note that complaints may result from other causes. These may include an illness contracted outside the building, acute sensitivity (e.g., allergies), job related stress or dissatisfaction, and other psychosocial factors. Nevertheless, studies show that symptoms may be caused or exacerbated by indoor air quality problems.

Causes of Sick Building Syndrome

A Word about Radon and Asbestos...

SBS and BRI are associated with acute or immediate health problems; radon and asbestos cause long-term diseases which occur years after exposure, and are therefore not considered to be among the causes of sick buildings. This is not to say that the latter are not serious health risks; both should be included in any comprehensive evaluation of a building's IAQ.

The following have been cited causes of or contributing factors to Sick Building Syndrome:

Inadequate ventilation: In the early and mid 1900's, building ventilation standards called for approximately 15 cubic feet per minute (cfm) of outside air for each building occupant, primarily to dilute and remove body odors. As a result of the 1973 oil embargo, however, national energy conservation measures called for a reduction in the amount of outdoor air provided for ventilation to 5 cfm per occupant. In many cases these reduced outdoor air ventilation rates were found to be inadequate to maintain the health and comfort of building occupants. Inadequate ventilation, which may also occur if heating, ventilating, and air conditioning (HVAC) systems do not effectively distribute air to people in the building, is thought to be an important factor in SBS. In an effort to achieve acceptable IAQ while minimizing energy consumption, the American Society of Heating, Refrigerating and Air-Conditioning Engineers (ASHRAE) recently revised its ventilation standard to provide a minimum of 15 cfm of outdoor air per person (20 cfm/person in office spaces). Up to 60 cfm/person may be required in some spaces (such as smoking lounges) depending on the activities that normally occur in that space (see ASHRAE Standard 62-1989).

Chemical contaminants from indoor sources: Most indoor air pollution comes from sources inside the building. For example, adhesives, carpeting, upholstery, manufactured wood products, copy machines, pesticides, and cleaning agents may emit volatile organic compounds (VOCs), including formaldehyde. Environmental tobacco smoke contributes high levels of VOCs, other toxic compounds, and respirable particulate matter. Research shows that some VOCs can cause chronic and acute health effects at high concentrations, and some are known carcinogens. Low to moderate levels of multiple VOCs may also produce acute reactions. Combustion products such as carbon monoxide, nitrogen dioxide, as well as respirable particles, can come from unvented kerosene and gas space heaters, wood stoves, fireplaces and gas stoves.

Chemical contaminants from outdoor sources: The outdoor air that enters a building can be a source of indoor air pollution. For example, pollutants from motor vehicle exhausts; plumbing vents, and building exhausts (e.g., bathrooms and kitchens) can enter the building through poorly located air intake vents, windows, and other openings. In addition, combustion products can enter a building from a nearby garage.

Biological contaminants: Bacteria, molds, pollen, and viruses are types of biological contaminants. These contaminants may breed in stagnant water that has accumulated in ducts, humidifiers and drain pans, or where water has collected on ceiling tiles, carpeting, or insulation. Sometimes insects or bird droppings can be a source of biological contaminants. Physical symptoms related to biological contamination include cough, chest tightness, fever, chills, muscle aches, and allergic responses such as mucous membrane irritation and upper respiratory congestion. One indoor bacterium, Legionella, has caused both Legionnaire's Disease and Pontiac Fever. These elements may act in combination, and may supplement other complaints such as inadequate temperature, humidity, or lighting. Even after a building investigation, however, the specific causes of the complaints may remain unknown.

Building Investigation Procedures

The goal of a building investigation is to identify and solve indoor air quality complaints in a way that prevents them from recurring and which avoids the creation of other problems. To achieve this goal, it is necessary for the investigator(s) to discover whether a complaint is actually related to indoor air quality, identify the cause of the complaint, and determine the most appropriate corrective actions.

An indoor air quality investigation procedure is best characterized as a cycle of information gathering, hypothesis formation, and hypothesis testing. It generally begins with a walk-through inspection of the problem area to provide information about the four basic factors that influence indoor air quality:

- The occupants
- The HVAC system

- Possible pollutant pathways
- Possible contaminant sources.

Preparation for a walk-through should include documenting easily obtainable information about the history of the building and of the complaints; identifying known HVAC zones and complaint areas; notifying occupants of the upcoming investigation; and, identifying key individuals needed for information and access. The walk-through itself entails visual inspection of critical building areas and consultation with occupants and staff.

The initial walk-through should allow the investigator to develop some possible explanations for the complaint. At this point, the investigator may have sufficient information to formulate a hypothesis, test the hypothesis, and see if the problem is solved. If it is, steps should be taken to ensure that it does not recur. However, if insufficient information is obtained from the walk through to construct a hypothesis, or if initial tests fail to reveal the problem, the investigator should move on to collect additional information to allow formulation of additional hypotheses. The process of formulating hypotheses, testing them, and evaluating them continues until the problem is solved.

Although air sampling for contaminants might seem to be the logical response to occupant complaints, it seldom provides information about possible causes. While certain basic measurements, e.g., temperature, relative humidity, CO_2, and air movement, can provide a useful "snapshot" of current building conditions, sampling for specific pollutant concentrations is often not required to solve the problem and can even be misleading. Contaminant concentration levels rarely exceed existing standards and guidelines even when occupants continue to report health complaints. Air sampling should not be undertaken until considerable information on the factors listed above has been collected, and any sampling strategy should be based on a comprehensive understanding of how the building operates and the nature of the complaints.

Solutions to Sick Building Syndrome

Solutions to Sick Building Syndrome usually include combinations of the following:

Pollutant source removal or modification is an effective approach to resolving an IAQ problem when sources are known and control is feasible. Examples include routine maintenance of HVAC systems, e.g., periodic cleaning or replacement of filters; replacement of water-stained ceiling tile and carpeting; institution of smoking restrictions; venting contaminant source emissions to the outdoors; storage and use of paints, adhesives, solvents, and pesticides in well ventilated areas, and use of these pollutant sources during periods of non-occupancy; and allowing time for building materials in new or remodelled areas to off-gas pollutants before occupancy. Several of these options may be exercised at one time.

Increasing ventilation rates and air distribution often can be a cost effective means of reducing indoor pollutant levels. HVAC systems should be designed, at a minimum, to meet ventilation standards in local building codes; however, many systems are not operated or maintained to ensure that these design ventilation rates are provided. In many buildings, IAQ can be improved by operating the HVAC system to at least its design standard, and to ASHRAE Standard 62-1989 if possible. When there are strong pollutant sources, local exhaust ventilation may be appropriate to exhaust contaminated air directly from the building. Local exhaust ventilation is particularly recommended to remove pollutants that accumulate in specific areas such as rest rooms, copy rooms, and printing facilities.

Air cleaning can be a useful adjunct to source control and ventilation but has certain limitations. Particle control devices such as the typical furnace filter are inexpensive but do not effectively capture small particles; high performance air filters capture the smaller, respirable particles but are relatively expensive to install and operate. Mechanical filters do not remove gaseous pollutants. Some specific gaseous pollutants may be removed by adsorbent beds, but these devices can be expensive and require frequent replacement of the adsorbent material. In sum, air cleaners can be useful, but have limited application.

Education and communication are important elements in both remedial and preventive indoor air quality management programs. When building occupants, management, and maintenance personnel fully communicate and understand the causes and consequences of IAQ problems, they can work more effectively together to prevent problems from occurring, or to solve them if they do.

Guidelines of US Environmental Protection Agency

Tour of Home–Living Room

A living room is usually a well-used area of a home and may harbour indoor pollutants. It is important to ventilate properly, keep second-hand smoke outside of the house, and vacuum and dust regularly.

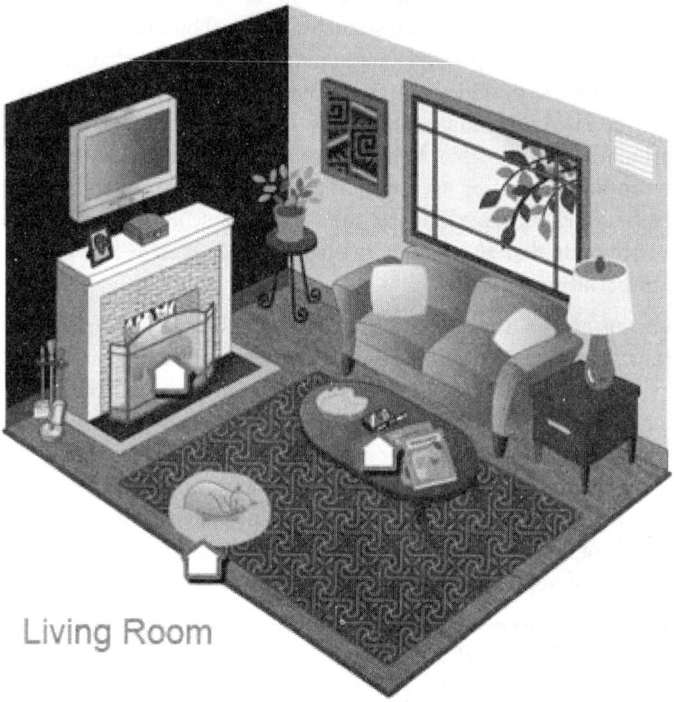

Pet Dander and Hair: Pets can trigger allergy and asthma attacks due to dander and hair. Keep them out of the sleeping areas, and away from upholstered furniture, carpets, and stuffed toys. Vacuum and clean carpets, rugs, and furniture often. Learn more at www.epa.gov/asthma/pets.html
Secondhand Smoke: Secondhand smoke from cigarettes, cigars, and other tobacco products can trigger asthma and other respiratory illnesses especially in children. To help protect children from secondhand smoke, do not smoke or allow others to smoke inside your home or car. Learn more at www.epa.gov/smokefree
Carbon Monoxide: Fireplaces and leaking chimneys are sources of carbon monoxide. Ventilate rooms that have fireplaces, make certain the flue damper is operational and fully open when in use, and ensure the chimney is properly sealed. Learn more at www.epa.gov/iaq/co.html

Bathroom

A bathroom is often the dampest area of a home. It is important to ventilate a bathroom during use and dry damp surfaces.

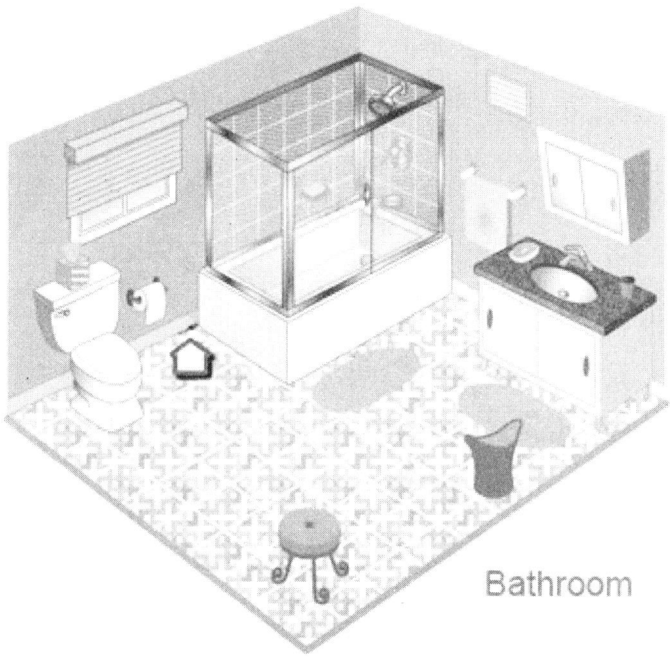

Mold: Bathrooms are a common source of mold. Humidity from showers can cause moisture problems, which will lead to mold growth. Mold can cause allergic reactions, asthma, and other respiratory ailments. Installing and using a ventilation fan will help to control moisture and inhibit mold growth. Learn more at www.epa.gov/mold

Bedroom

A bedroom often contains materials that collect dust. It is important to clean bedding and other fabrics, and vacuum regularly.

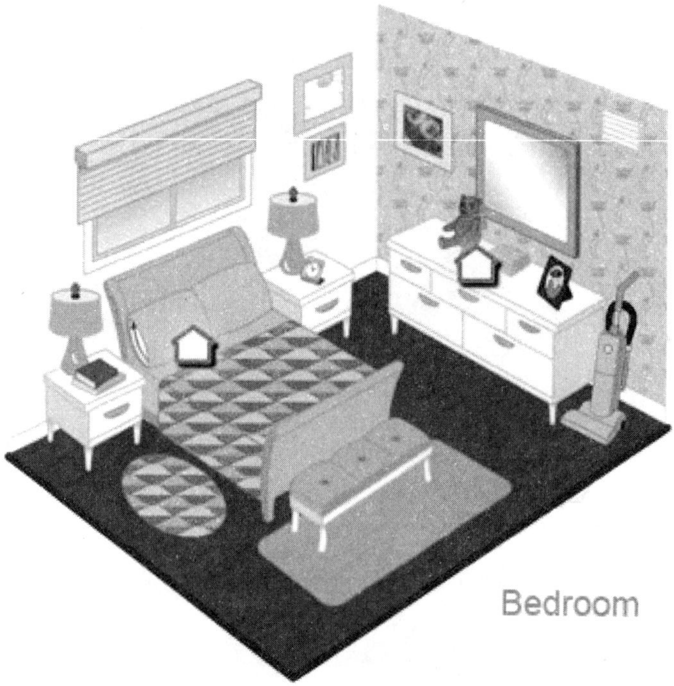

Dust: Dust mites can trigger allergy and asthma attacks. Dust mites are everywhere especially on pillows, blankets, carpets, upholstered furniture, and stuffed toys Dust and vacuum your home regularly, wash bedding, and use allergen-proof mattress and pillow covers. Learn more at www.epa.gov/asthma/dustmites.html

Kitchen

A kitchen has appliances that may leak gases, and often contain chemicals for cleaning or removing pests. It is important to properly maintain and ventilate appliances, and safely store chemicals.

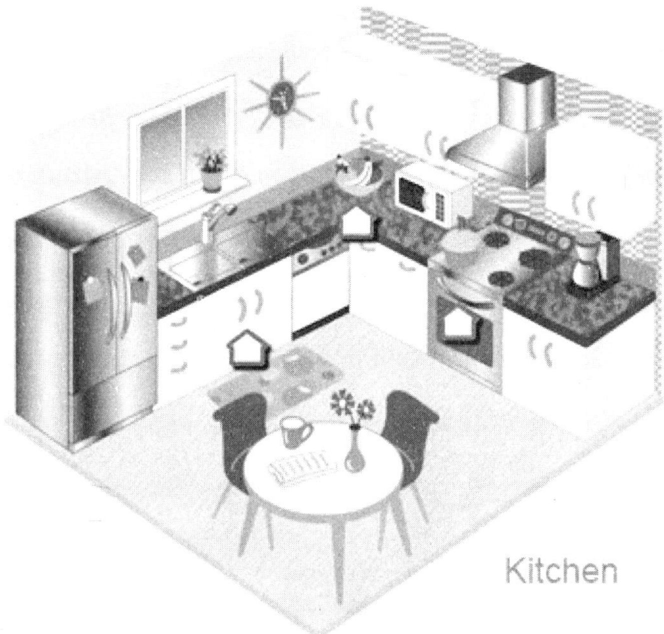

Pesticides: Pesticides, used to rid homes of rodents, termites, insects, and other pests, can irritate the eyes, nose, and throat; damage the central nervous system and kidneys; and increase the risk of cancer. Don't leave food out, and if you must use pesticides, ventilate during and after use and follow directions to limit exposure. Use non-chemical methods of pest control when possible. Learn more at www.epa.gov/iaq/pesticid.html
Volatile Organic Compounds (VOCs): Common household cleaners, often placed under the kitchen sink, release Volatile Organic Compounds (VOCs), when used and stored. Store household products that contain chemicals according to manufacturers' instructions and keep all products away from children. Consider purchasing cleaners without VOCs. Learn more at www.epa.gov/iaq/voc.html
Carbon Monoxide: To help prevent carbon monoxide exposure, make sure appliances such as gas stoves vent to the outside whenever possible and that all appliances are properly installed, used, and maintained. Learn more at www.epa.gov/iaq/co.html

Basement

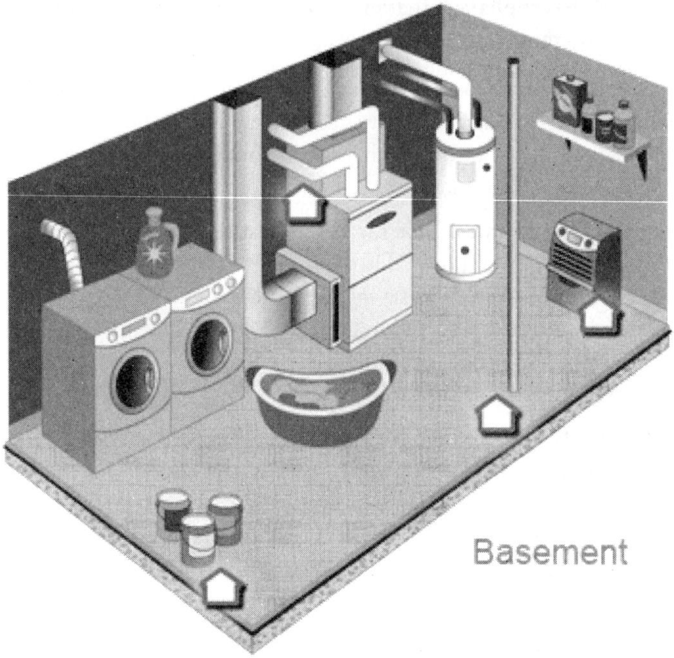

A basement is a source of air leaks and moisture, and often contains various chemicals. It is important to ventilate, seal cracks, and properly store all chemicals.

Carbon Monoxide

Combustion heating and cooling appliances such as heating, ventilation, and air conditioning units, gasoline-powered heaters, and other appliances are sources of carbon monoxide. Properly install, use, and maintain fuel-burning appliances. Install carbon monoxide detectors in living spaces. Learn more at www.epa.gov/iaq/co.html

Volatile Organic Compounds (VOCs)

Paints, resins, paint thinners, and chemicals, and other products, will still release Volatile Organic Compounds (VOCs) even while stored properly. Make sure there is plenty of ventilation when painting, remodeling, or using other products that may release VOCs. Consider purchasing low and no VOC products. Learn more at www.epa.gov/iaq/voc.html

Mold

Basements can be damp. Install a properly sized dehumidifier to help keep your basement at an appropriate humidity level and reduce the potential for mold. It is important to dry water-damaged areas and items within 24-48 hours to prevent mold growth. Learn more at www.epa.gov/mold

Radon

Radon is the leading cause of lung cancer among non-smokers in the U.S. It is a naturally occurring radioactive gas that can enter a home through cracks and openings in floors and walls that are in contact with the ground. Testing your home is simple and inexpensive. Learn more at www.epa.gov/radon

- **For Existing Homes:** Test for radon–testing is the only way to know if radon is in your home. Do-it-yourself test kits are convenient and accessible, or you may choose to have a professional test your home. If the test result indicates your radon level is too high, a qualified radon service professional can install a radon mitigation system. Find a qualified radon service professional at www.epa.gov/radon/radontest.html
- **For New Construction:** Radon-resistant new construction (RRNC) draws radon from the soil and vents it through a pipe to the roof, preventing its entry into the house. This technique uses common materials and building skills. RRNC costs less than retrofitting a similar radon reduction system after the house is finished. New home buyers should ask their build to include RRNC features. All new homes, even new RRNC ones, should be tested for radon. Learn more at www.epa.gov/radon/rrnc

Guidelines by Environmental Illness Resource on Multiple Chemical Sensitivity

An Overview

Multiple Chemical Sensitivity is the name given to a syndrome in which a sufferer experiences multiple symptoms upon exposure to minute amounts of everyday chemicals. There is currently no officially recognized definition for Multiple Chemical Sensitivity. This is due to the fact that very little is known about it, especially the mechanisms involved with the onset of symptoms. Leading theories suggest a possible role for a hypersensitive central nervous system, immune dysfunction and impaired detoxification by liver enzymes. Some medical professionals, and even organizations, continue to insist that the syndrome is psychological in origin, even in the face of a growing amount of evidence from studies that show clear abnormalities in people with MCS on exposure to normally safe levels of chemicals. Through 1999 there were a total of 618 scientific articles, editorials, books, book chapters and reports relating to MCS. Of these, 308 supported an organic/physiological basis for symptoms whereas only 137 supported a psychological interpretation. (Source: www.mcsrr.org).

Although there is no definition universally accepted by the established medical institutions, Multiple Chemical Sensitivity experts (Bartha *et al* 1999) have come to a consensus on the criteria for diagnosis, and thus far these criteria remain unrefuted in the published literature. These criteria are as follows:

- The symptoms are reproducible with [repeated chemical] exposure.
- The condition is chronic.
- Low levels of exposure [lower than previously or commonly tolerated] result in manifestations of the syndrome.
- The symptoms improve or resolve when the incitants are removed.
- Responses occur to multiple chemically unrelated substances.
- Symptoms involve multiple organ systems [Added in 1999].

It's reasonable to expect that these criteria will be officially adopted in a form very close to the above in the relatively near future.

To complicate matters, however, a number of influential medical institutions, such as the American Academy of Allergy Asthma and Immunology (AAAAI), have renamed the illness as 'Idiopathic Environmental Intolerance' (IEI). They cite the reason for this to be the fact that no immune system involvement has been proven thus far and since "sensitivity" in medical jargon technically refers to an immune reaction, they deem MCS to be inaccurate. For the general population "sensitivity" and "intolerance" generally mean the same thing and MCS is so well known that most people are sticking with this name for now.

Symptoms

Many MCS sufferers can trace the start of their illness to an acute exposure to highly toxic chemicals (Gulf War veterans, and farmers using pesticides for example). For other sufferers the illness develops over a long period of time most likely involving chronic low level exposure to chemical substances. Although MCS can occur on its own, a large number of sufferers also suffer from CFS, Fibromyalgia and other related disorders. This obviously points to the possibility that all these illnesses are part of the same underlying process and likely have common causes.

MCS is a chronic condition with the patient usually experiencing some level of unwellness all the time. However, patients have an acute reaction when exposed to minute amounts of the chemicals to which they are sensitive. Often the level of a chemical that triggers a reaction may be so low that the sufferer can't even smell it.

Common symptoms of MCS upon exposure:

- Fatigue
- Headaches
- Disorientation
- Dizziness and Faintness
- Flu-like symptoms
- Nausea
- Irregular or Rapid Heartbeat
- Muscle and Joint Pain
- Gastrointestinal problems
- Mood Disturbances-Depression/Anxiety/Irritability
- Short-term Memory Problems
- Asthma/Breathing Problems
- Rashes

Most sufferers have a distinct reaction upon every exposure. It is common to first experience dizziness, disorientation, rapid heartbeat and mood changes followed by flu-like illness and muscle/joint aches. In severe cases, the flu-like illness and aching can persist for days.

Guidelines by United States Consumer Product Safety Commission

An Update On Formaldehyde: 1997 Revision

CPSC Document #725

What is Formaldehyde?

Formaldehyde is an important industrial chemical used to make other chemicals, building materials, and household products. It is one of the large family of chemical compounds called volatile organic compounds or "VOCs". The term volatile means that the compounds vaporize, that is, become a gas, at normal room temperatures. Formaldehyde serves many purposes in products. It is used as a part of:

- The glue or adhesive in pressed wood products (particleboard, hardwood plywood, and medium density fibreboard (MDF));
- Preservatives in some paints, coatings, and cosmetics;
- The coating that provides permanent press quality to fabrics and draperies;
- The finish used to coat paper products; and
- Certain insulation materials (urea-formaldehyde foam and fibreglass insulation).

Formaldehyde is released into the air by burning wood, kerosene or natural gas, by automobiles, and by cigarettes. Formaldehyde can off-gas from materials made with it. It is also a naturally occurring substance.

The U.S. Consumer Safety Commission has produced this booklet to tell you about formaldehyde found in the indoor air. This booklet tells you where you may come in contact with formaldehyde, how it may affect your health, and how you might reduce your exposure to it.

Why Should You Be Concerned?

Formaldehyde is a colourless, strong-smelling gas. When present in the air at levels above 0.1 ppm (parts in a million parts of air), it can cause watery eyes, burning sensations in the eyes, nose and throat, nausea, coughing, chest tightness, wheezing, skin rashes, and allergic reactions. It also has been observed to cause cancer in scientific studies using laboratory animals and may cause cancer in humans. Typical exposures to humans are much lower; thus any risk of causing cancer is believed to be small at the level at which humans are exposed.

Formaldehyde can affect people differently. Some people are very sensitive to formaldehyde while others may not have any noticeable reaction to the same level.

Persons have developed allergic reactions (allergic skin disease and hives) to formaldehyde through skin contact with solutions of formaldehyde or durable-press clothing containing formaldehyde. Others have developed asthmatic reactions and skin rashes from exposure to formaldehyde.

Formaldehyde is just one of several gases present indoors that may cause illnesses. Many of these gases, as well as colds and flu, cause similar symptoms.

What Levels of Formaldehyde Are Normal?

Formaldehyde is normally present at low levels, usually less than 0.03 ppm, in both outdoor and indoor air. The outdoor air in rural areas has lower concentrations while urban areas have higher concentrations. Residences or offices that contain products that release formaldehyde to the air can have formaldehyde levels of greater than 0.03 ppm. Products that may add formaldehyde to the air include particleboard used as flooring under layment, shelving, furniture and cabinets; MDF in cabinets and furniture; hardwood plywood wall panels, and urea-formaldehyde foam used as insulation. As formaldehyde levels increase, illness or discomfort is more likely to occur and may be more serious.

Efforts have been made by both the government and industry to reduce exposure to formaldehyde. CPSC voted to ban urea-formaldehyde foam insulation in 1982. That ban was over-turned in the courts, but this action greatly reduced the residential use of the insulation product. CPSC, the Department of Housing and Urban Development (HUD) and other federal agencies have historically worked with the pressed wood industry to further reduce the release of the chemical from their products. A 1985 HUD regulation covering the use of pressed wood products in manufactured housing was designed to ensure that indoor levels are below 0.4 ppm. However, it would be unrealistic to expect to completely remove formaldehyde from the air. Some persons who are extremely sensitive to formaldehyde may need to reduce or stop using these products.

What Affects Formaldehyde Levels?

Formaldehyde levels in the indoor air depend mainly on what is releasing the formaldehyde (the source), the temperature, the humidity, and the air exchange rate (the amount of outdoor air entering or leaving the indoor area). Increasing the flow of outdoor air to the inside decreases the formaldehyde levels. Decreasing this flow of outdoor air by sealing the residence or office increases the formaldehyde level in the indoor air.

As the temperature rises, more formaldehyde is emitted from the product. The reverse is also true; less formaldehyde is emitted at lower temperature. Humidity also affects the release of formaldehyde from the product. As humidity rises more formaldehyde is released.

The formaldehyde levels in a residence change with the season and from day-to-day and day-to-night. Levels may be high on a hot and humid day and low on a cool, dry day. Understanding these factors is important when you consider measuring the levels of formaldehyde.

Some sources-such as pressed wood products containing urea-formaldehyde glues, urea-formaldehyde foam insulation, durable-press fabrics, and draperies-release more formaldehyde when new. As they age, the formaldehyde release decreases.

What are the Major Sources?

1. Urea-formaldehyde foam insulation: During the 1970s, many homeowners installed this insulation to save energy. Many of these homes had high levels of formaldehyde soon afterwards. Sale of urea-formaldehyde foam insulation has largely stopped. Formaldehyde released from this product decreases rapidly after the first few months and reaches background levels in a few years. Therefore, urea-formaldehyde foam insulation installed 5 to 10 years ago is unlikely to still release formaldehyde.

2. Durable-press fabrics, draperies and coated paper products: In the early 1960s, there were several reports of allergic reactions to formaldehyde from durable-press fabrics and coated paper products. Such reports have declined in recent years as industry has taken steps to reduce formaldehyde levels. Draperies made of formaldehyde-treated durable press fabrics may add slightly to indoor formaldehyde levels.

3. Cosmetics, paints, coatings, and some wet-strength paper products: The amount of formaldehyde present in these products is small and is of slight concern. However, persons sensitive to formaldehyde may have allergic reactions.

4. Pressed wood products: Pressed wood products, especially those containing urea-formaldehyde glues, are a source of formaldehyde. These products include particleboard used as flooring under layment, shelves, cabinets, and furniture; hardwood plywood wall panels; and medium density fibreboard used in drawers, cabinets and furniture. When the surfaces and edges of these products are unlaminated or uncoated they have the potential to release more formaldehyde. Manufacturers have reduced formaldehyde emissions from pressed wood products by 80-90% from the levels of the early 1980Õs.

5. Combustion sources: Burning materials such as wood, kerosene, cigarettes and natural gas, and operating internal combustion engines (e.g. automobiles), produce small quantities of formaldehyde. Combustion sources add small amounts of formaldehyde to indoor air.

6. Products such as carpets or gypsum board do not contain significant amounts of formaldehyde when new. They may trap formaldehyde emitted from other sources and later release the formaldehyde into the indoor air when the temperature and humidity change.

Do You Have Formaldehyde-Related Symptoms?

There are several formaldehyde-related symptoms, such as watery eyes, runny nose, burning sensation in the eyes, nose, and throat, headaches and fatigue. These symptoms may also occur because of the common cold, the flu or other pollutants that may be present in the indoor air. If these symptoms lessen when you are away from home or office but reappear upon your return, they may be caused by indoor pollutants, including formaldehyde. Examine your environment. Have you recently moved into a new or different home or office? Have you recently remodelled or installed new cabinets or furniture? Symptoms may be due to formaldehyde exposure. You should contact your physician and/or state or local health department for help. Your physician can help to determine if the cause of your symptoms is formaldehyde or other pollutants.

Should You Measure Formaldehyde?

Only trained professionals should measure formaldehyde because they know how to interpret the results. If you become ill, and the illness persists following the purchase of furniture or remodelling with pressed wood products, you might not need to measure formaldehyde. Since these are possible sources, you can take action. You may become ill after painting, sealing, making repairs, and/or applying pest control treatment in your home or office. In such cases, indoor air pollutants other than formaldehyde may be the cause. If the source is not obvious, you should consult a physician to determine whether or not your symptoms might relate to indoor air quality problems. If your physician believes that you may be sensitive to formaldehyde, you may want to make some measurements. As discussed earlier, many factors can affect the level of formaldehyde on a given day in an office or residence. This is why a professional is best suited to make an accurate measurement of the levels.

Do-it-yourself formaldehyde measuring devices are available, however these devices can only provide a "ball park" estimate for the formaldehyde level in the area. If you use such a device, carefully follow the instructions.

How Do You Reduce Formaldehyde Exposure?

Every day you probably use many products that contain formaldehyde. You may not be able to avoid coming in contact with some formaldehyde in your normal daily routine. If you are sensitive to formaldehyde, you will need to avoid many everyday items to reduce symptoms. For most people, a low-level exposure to formaldehyde (up to 0.1 ppm) does not produce symptoms. People who suspect they are sensitive to formaldehyde should work closely with a knowledgeable physician to make sure that it is formaldehyde causing their symptoms.

You can avoid exposure to higher levels by:

- Purchasing pressed wood products such as particleboard, MDF, or hardwood plywood for construction or remodeling of homes, or for do-it-yourself projects, that are labeled or stamped to be in conformance with American National Standards Institute (ANSI) criteria. Particleboard should be in conformance with ANSI A208.1-1993. For particleboard flooring, look for ANSI grades "PBU", "D2", or "D3" actually stamped on the panel. MDF should be in conformance with ANSI A208.2-1994; and hardwood plywood with ANSI/HPVA HP-1-1994. These standards all specify lower formaldehyde emission levels.
- Purchasing furniture or cabinets that contain a high percentage of panel surface and edges that are laminated or coated. Unlaminated or uncoated (raw) panels of pressed wood products will generally emit more formaldehyde than those that are laminated or coated.
- Using alternative products such as wood panel products not made with urea-formaldehyde glues, lumber or metal.
- Avoiding the use of foamed-in-place insulation containing formaldehyde, especially urea-formaldehyde foam insulation.
- Washing durable-press fabrics before use.

How Do You Reduce Existing Formaldehyde Levels?

The choice of methods to reduce formaldehyde is unique to your situation. People who can help you select appropriate methods are your state or local health department, physician, or professional expert in indoor air problems. Here are some of the methods to reduce indoor levels of formaldehyde.

1. Bring large amounts of fresh air into the home. Increase ventilation by opening doors and windows and installing an exhaust fan(s).
2. Seal the surfaces of the formaldehyde-containing products that are not already laminated or coated. You may use a vapour barrier such as some paints, varnishes, or a layer of vinyl or polyurethane-like materials. Be sure to seal completely, with a material that does not itself contain formaldehyde. Many paints and coatings will emit other VOCs when curing, so be sure to ventilate the area well during and after treatment.
3. Remove from your home the product that is releasing formaldehyde in the indoor air. When other materials in the area such as carpets, gypsum boards, etc., have absorbed formaldehyde, these products may also start releasing it into the air. Overall levels of formaldehyde can be lower if you increase the ventilation over an extended period.

One method NOT recommended by CPSC is a chemical treatment with strong ammonia (28-29% ammonia in water) which results in a temporary decrease in formaldehyde levels. We strongly discourage such treatment since ammonia in this strength is extremely dangerous to handle. Ammonia may damage the brass fittings of a natural gas system, adding a fire and explosion danger.

Guidelines by Consumer Product Safety Commission

Biological Pollutants in Your Home

CPSC Document #425

This booklet will help you understand:

1. What indoor biological pollution is
2. Whether your home or lifestyle promotes its development
3. How to control its growth and build-up

Outdoor air pollution in cities is a major health problem. Much effort and money continues to be spent cleaning up pollution in the outdoor air. But air pollution can be a problem where you least expect it, in the place you may have thought was safest -- your home. Many ordinary activities such as cooking, heating, cooling, cleaning, and redecorating can cause the release and spread of indoor pollutants at home. Studies have shown that the air in our homes can be even more polluted than outdoor air.

Many Americans spend up to 90 percent of their time indoors, often at home. Therefore, breathing clean indoor air can have an important impact on health. People who are inside a great deal may be at greater risk of developing health problems, or having problems made worse by indoor air pollutants. These people include infants, young children the elderly and those with chronic illnesses.

What Are Biological Pollutants?

Biological pollutants are or were living organisms. They promote poor indoor air quality and may be a major cause of days lost from work or school, and of doctor and hospital visits. Some can even damage surfaces inside and outside your house. Biological pollutants can travel through the air and are often invisible.

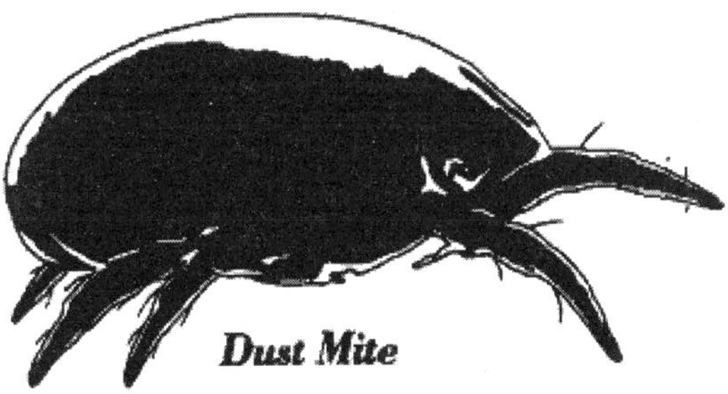

Dust mites are microscopic - this drawing has been enlarged to show detail.

Dust mites are microscopic - this drawing has been enlarged to show detail

Some common indoor biological pollutants are:

- Animal Dander (minute scales from hair, feathers, or skin)
- Dust Mite and Cockroach parts
- Infectious agents (bacteria or viruses)
- Pollen

Some of these substances are in every home. It is impossible to get rid of them all. Even a spotless home may permit the growth of biological pollutants. Two conditions are essential to support biological growth nutrients and moisture. These conditions can be found in many locations, such as bathrooms, damp or flooded basements, wet appliances (such as humidifiers or air conditioners), and even some carpets and furniture.

Modern materials and construction techniques may reduce the amount of outside air brought into buildings which may result in high moisture levels inside. Using humidifiers, unvented heaters, and air conditioners in our homes has increased the chances of moisture forming on interior surfaces. This encourages the growth of certain biological pollutants.

The Scope Of The Problem:

Most information about sources and health effects of biological pollutants is based on studies of large office buildings and two surveys of homes in northern U.S. and Canada. These surveys show that 30% to 50% of all structures have damp conditions which may encourage the growth and buildup of biological pollutants. This percentage is likely to be higher in warm, moist climates. Some diseases or illnesses have been linked with biological pollutants in the indoor environment. However, many of them also have causes unrelated to the indoor environment. Therefore, we do nut know how many health problems relate only to poor indoor air.

Health Effects Of Biological Pollutants:

All of us are exposed to biological pollutants. However, the effects on our health depend upon the type and amount of biological pollution and the individual person. Some people do not experience health reactions from certain biological pollutants, while others may experience one or more of the following reactions:

- Allergic
- Infectious
- Toxic

Except for the spread of infections indoors, ALLERGIC REACTIONS may be the most common health problem with indoor air quality in homes. They are often connected with animal dander (mostly from cats and dogs), with house dust mites (microscopic animals living in household dust), and with pollen. Allergic reactions can range from mildly uncomfortable to life-threatening, as in a severe asthma attack. Some common signs and symptoms are:

- Watery eyes
- Runny nose and sneezing
- Nasal congestion
- Itching
- Fatigue
- Coughing
- Wheezing and difficulty breathing
- Headache

Health experts are especially concerned about people with asthma These people have very sensitive airways that can react to various irritants, making breathing difficult. The number of people who have asthma has greatly increased in recent years. The number of people with asthma has gone up by 59 percent since 1970, to a total of 9.6 million people. Asthma in children under 15 years of age has increased 41 percent in the same period, to a total of 2.6 million children. The number of deaths from asthma is up by 68 percent since 1979, to a total of almost 4,400 deaths per year.

Talking to Your Doctor:

Are you concerned about the effects on your health that may be related to biological pollutants in your home? Before you discuss your concerns with your doctor, you should know the answers to the following questions. This information can help the doctor determine whether your health problems may be related to biological pollution.

Does anyone in the family have frequent headaches, fevers, itchy watery eyes, a stuffy nose, dry throat, or a cough? Does anyone complain of feeling tired or dizzy all the time? Is anyone wheezing or having difficulties breathing on a regular basis?

Did these symptoms appear after you moved to a new or different home?

Do the symptoms disappear when you go to school or the office or go away on a trip, and return when you come back?

Have you recently remodelled your home or done any energy conservation work, such as installing insulation, storm windows, or weather stripping? Did your symptoms occur during or after these activities?

Does your home feel humid? Can you see moisture on the windows or on other surfaces, such as walls and ceilings?

What is the usual temperature in your home? Is it very hot or cold?

Have you recently had water damage?

Is your basement wet or damp?

Is there any obvious mold or mildew?

Does any part of your home have a musty or moldy odor?

Is the air stale?

Do you have pets?

Do your house plants show signs of mold?

Do you have air conditioners or humidifiers that have not been properly cleaned?

Does your home have cockroaches or rodents?

INFECTIOUS DISEASES caused by bacteria and viruses, such as flu, measles, chicken pox, and tuberculosis, may be spread indoors. Most infectious diseases pass from person to person through physical contact. Crowded conditions with poor air circulation can promote this spread. Some bacteria and viruses thrive in buildings and circulate through indoor ventilation systems. For example, the bacterium causing Legionnaire's disease, a serious and sometimes lethal infection, and Pontiac Fever, a flu-like illness, have circulated in some large buildings.

TOXIC REACTIONS are the least studied and understood health problem caused by some biological air pollutants in the home. Toxins can damage a variety of organs and tissues in the body, including the liver, the central nervous system, the digestive tract, and the immune system.

Coping With the Problem

Checking Your Home:

There is no simple and cheap way to sample the air in your home to determine the level of all biological pollutants. Experts suggest that sampling for biological pollutants is not a useful problem-solving tool. Even if you had your home tested, it is almost impossible to know which biological pollutant(s) cause various symptoms or health problems. The amount of most biological substances required to cause disease is unknown and varies from one person to the next.

Does this make the problem sound hopeless? On the contrary, you can take several simple, practical actions to help remove sources of biological pollutants, to help get rid of pollutants, and to prevent their return.

Self-Inspection: A Walk Through Your Home:

Begin by touring your household. Follow your nose, and use your eyes. Two major factors help create conditions for biological pollutants to grow nutrients and constant moisture with poor air circulation.

Dust and construction materials, such as wood, wall-board, and insulation, contain nutrients that allow biological pollutants to grow. Firewood also is a source of moisture, fungi, and bugs.

Appliances such as humidifiers, kerosene and gas heaters, and gas stoves add moisture to the air.

A musty odour, moisture on hard surfaces, or even water stains, may be caused by:

- Air-conditioning units
- Basements, attics, and crawlspaces
- Bathrooms
- Carpets
- Heating and air-conditioning ducts
- Humidifiers and dehumidifiers
- Refrigerator drip pans

What You Can Do About Biological Pollutants:

Before you give away the family pet or move, there are less drastic steps that can be taken to reduce potential problems. Properly cleaning and maintaining your home can help reduce the problem and may avoid interrupting your normal routine. People who have health problems such as asthma, or are allergic, may need to do this and more. Discuss this with your doctor.

Moisture Control:

Water in your home can come from many sources. Water can enter your home by leaking or by seeping through basement floors. Showers or even cooking can add moisture to the air in your home. The amount of moisture that the air in your home can hold depends on the temperature of the air. As the temperature goes down, the air is able to hold less moisture. This is why, in cold weather, moisture condenses on cold surfaces (for example, drops of water form on the inside of a window). This moisture can encourage biological pollutants to grow.

There are many ways to control moisture in your home:

Fix leaks and seepage. If water is entering the house from the outside, your options range from simple landscaping to extensive excavation and waterproofing. (The ground should slope away from the house). Water in the basement can result from the lack of gutters or a water flow toward the house. Water leaks in pipes or around tubs and sinks can provide a place for biological pollutants to grow.

Put a plastic cover over dirt crawlspaces to prevent moisture from coming in from the ground. Be sure crawlspaces are well-ventilated.

Use exhaust fans in bathrooms and kitchens to remove moisture to the outside (not into the attic).

Vent your clothes dryer to the outside.

Turn off certain appliances (such as humidifiers or kerosene heaters) if you notice moisture on windows and other surfaces.

Use dehumidifiers and air conditioners, especially in hot, humid climates, to reduce moisture in the air, but be sure that the appliances themselves don't become sources of biological pollutants.

Raise the temperature of cold surfaces where moisture condenses. Use insulation or storm windows. (A storm window installed on the inside works better than one installed on the outside) Open doors between rooms (especially doors to closets which may be colder than the rooms) to increase circulation. Circulation carries heat to the cold surfaces Increase air circulation by using fans and by moving furniture from wall corners to promote air and heat circulation. Be sure that your house has a source of fresh air and can expel excessive moisture from the home.

Pay special attention to carpet on concrete floors. Carpet can absorb moisture and serve as a place for biological pollutants to grow. Use area rugs which can be taken up and washed often In certain climates, if carpet is to be installed over a concrete floor, it maybe necessary to use a vapour barrier (plastic sheeting) over the concrete and cover that with sub-flooring (insulation covered with plywood) to prevent a moisture problem.

Moisture problems and their solutions differ from one climate to another. The Northeast is cold and wet, the Southwest is hot and dry, the South is hot and wet, and the Western Mountain states are cold and dry. All of these regions can have moisture problems. For example, evaporative coolers used in the Southwest can encourage the growth of biological pollutants. In other hot regions, the use of air conditioners which cool the air too quickly may prevent the air conditioners from running long enough to remove excess moisture from the air. The types of construction and weatherization for the different climates can lead to different problems and solutions.

Where Biological Pollutants May Be Found in the Home

1. Dirty air conditioners
2. Dirty humidifiers and/or dehumidifiers
3. Bathroom without vents or windows
4. Kitchen without vents or windows
5. Dirty refrigerator drip pans
6. Laundry room with unvented dryer
7. Unventilated attic
8. Carpet on damp basement floor
9. Bedding
10. Closet on outside wall
11. Dirty heating/air conditioning system
12. Dogs or cats
13. Water damage (around windows, the roof or the basement)

Maintain and clean all appliances that come in contact with water.

Have major appliances, such as furnaces, heat pumps and central air conditioners, inspected and cleaned regularly by a professional, especially before seasonal use. Change filters on heating and cooling systems according to manufacturer's directions. (In general, change filters monthly during use.) When first turning on the heating or air conditioning at the start of the season, consider leaving your home until it airs out.

Have window or wall air-conditioning units cleaned and serviced regularly by a professional, especially before the cooling season. Air conditioners can help reduce the entry of allergy-causing pollen. But they may also become a source of biological pollutants if not properly maintained. Clean the coils and rinse the drain pans according to manufacturer's instructions, so water cannot collect in pools.

Have furnace-attached humidifiers cleaned and serviced regularly by a professional, especially before the heating season.

Follow manufacturer's instructions when using any type of humidifier Experts differ on the benefits of using humidifiers. If you do use a portable humidifier (approximately 1 to 2 gallon tanks), be sure to empty its tank every day and refill with distilled or de-mineralized water, or even fresh tap water if the other types of water are unavailable For larger portable humidifiers, change the water as recommended by the manufacturer. Unplug the appliance before cleaning. Every third day, clean all surfaces coming in contact with

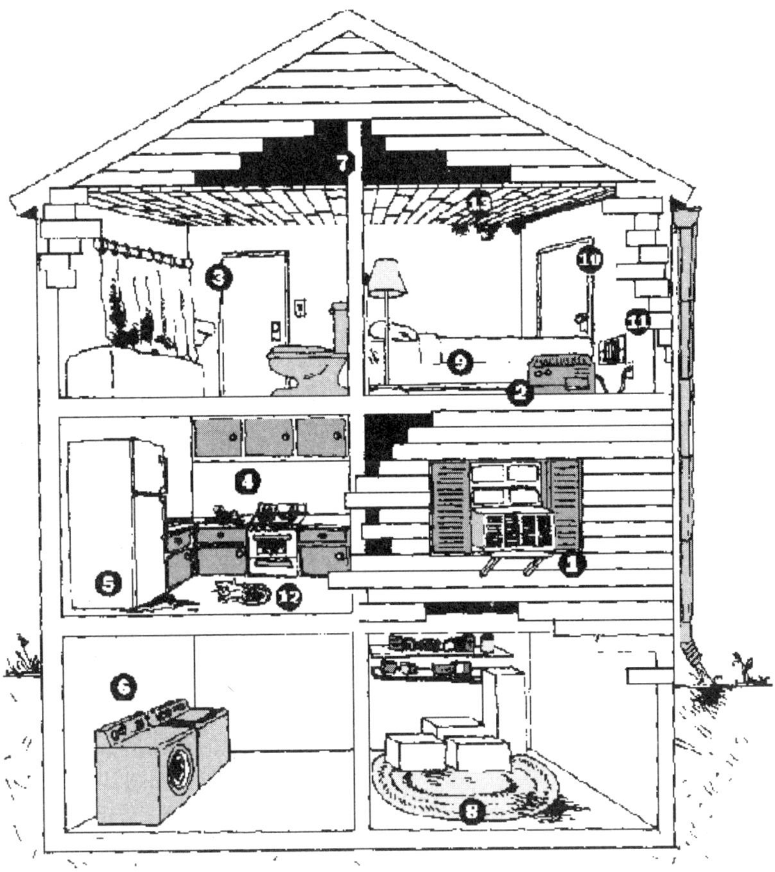

water with a 3% solution of hydrogen peroxide, using a brush to loosen deposits Some manufacturers recommend using diluted household bleach for cleaning and maintenance, generally in a solution of one-half cup bleach to one gallon water When any household chemical, rinse well to remove all traces of chemical before refilling humidifier.

Empty dehumidifiers daily and clean often. If possible, have the appliance drip directly into a drain. Follow manufacturer's instructions for cleaning and maintenance. Always disconnect the appliance before cleaning.

Clean refrigerator drip pans regularly according to manufacturer's instructions. If refrigerator and freezer doors don't seal properly, moisture may build up and mold can grow. Remove any mold on door gaskets and replace faulty gaskets.

Clean Surfaces

Clean moist surfaces, such as showers and kitchen counters.

Remove mold from walls, ceilings, floors, and panelling. Do not simply cover mold with paint, stain, varnish, or a moisture-proof sealer, as it may resurface.

Replace moldy shower curtains, or remove them and scrub well with a household cleaner and rinse before rehanging them.

Dust Control

Controlling dust is very important for people who are allergic to animal dander and mites. You cannot see mites, but you can either remove their favourite breeding grounds or keep these areas dry and clean. Dust mites can thrive in sofas, stuffed chairs, carpets, and bedding. Open shelves, fabric wallpaper, knick-knacks, and venetian blinds are also sources of dust mites. Dust mites live deep in the carpet and are not removed by vacuuming. Many doctors suggest that their mite-allergic patients use washable area rugs rather than wall-to-wall carpet.

Always wash bedding in hot water (at least 130° F) to kill dust mites. Cold water won't do the job. Launder bedding at least every 7 to 10 days.

Use synthetic or foam rubber mattress pads and pillows, and plastic mattress covers if you are allergic Do not use fuzzy wool blankets, feather or wool-stuffed comforters, and feather pillows.

Clean rooms and closets well, dust and vacuum often to remove surface dust. Vacuuming and other cleaning may not remove all animal dander, dust mite material, and other biological pollutants. Some particles are so small they can pass through vacuum bags and remain in the air If you are allergic to dust, wear a mask when vacuuming or dusting. People who are highly allergy-prone should not perform these tasks. They may even need to leave the house when someone else is cleaning.

Before You Move

Protect yourself by inspecting your potential new home. If you identify problems, have the landlord or seller correct them before you move in, or even consider moving elsewhere.

Have professionals check the heating and cooling system, including humidifiers and vents Have duct lining and insulation checked for growth.

Check for exhaust fans in bathrooms and kitchens If there are no vents, do the kitchen and bathrooms have at least one window a piece? Does the cook top have a hood vented outside?

Does the clothes dryer vent outside? Are all vents to the outside of the building, not in attics or crawlspaces?

Look for obvious mold growth throughout the house, including attics, basements, and crawlspaces and around the foundation. See if there are many plants close to the house, particularly if they are damp and rotting. They are a potential source of biological pollutants. Downspouts from roof gutters should route water away from the building.

Look for stains on the walls, floor or carpet (including any carpet over concrete floors) as evidence of previous flooding or moisture problems. Is there moisture on windows and surfaces? Are there signs of leaks or seepage in the basement?

Look for rotted building materials which may suggest moisture or water damage.

If you or anyone else in the family has a pet allergy, ask if any pets have lived in the home.

Examine the design of the building. Remember that in cold climates, overhanging areas, rooms over unheated garages, and closets on outside walls may be prone to problems with biological pollutants.

Look for signs of cockroaches.

Warning!

Carefully read instructions for use and any cautionary labeling on cleaning products before beginning cleaning procedures.

Do not mix any chemical products. Especially, never mix cleaners containing bleach with any product (such as ammonia) which does not have instructions for such mixing When chemicals are combined, a dangerous gas can sometimes be formed.

Household chemicals may cause burning or irritation to skin and eyes.

Household chemicals may be harmful if swallowed, or inhaled.

Avoid contact with skin, eyes, mucous membranes and clothing.

Avoid breathing vapour. Open all windows and doors and use an exhaust fan that sends the air outside.

Keep household chemicals out of reach of children.

Rinse treated surface areas well to remove all traces of chemicals.

Correcting Water Damage

What if damage is already done? Follow these guidelines for correcting water damage:

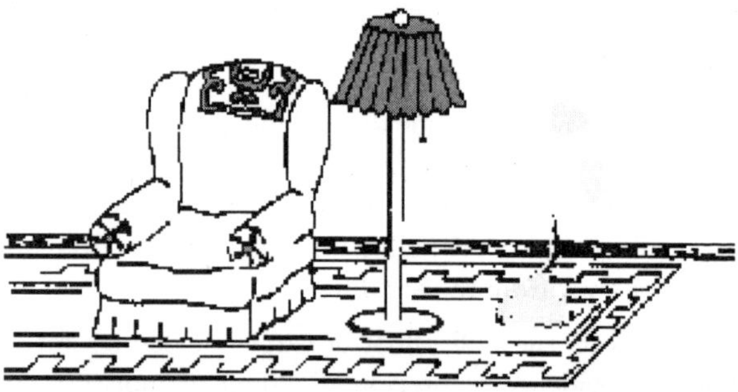

Throw out mattresses, wicker furniture, straw baskets and the like that have been water damaged or contain mold. These cannot be recovered.

Discard any water-damaged furnishings such as carpets, drapes, stuffed toys, upholstered furniture and ceiling tales, unless they can be recovered by steam cleaning or hot water washing and thorough drying.

Remove and replace wet insulation to prevent conditions where biological pollutants can grow.

Guidelines by Consumer Product Safety Commission

What You Should Know About Using Paint Strippers

CPSC Document #423

If not properly used, paint strippers are hazardous to your health and safety

Paint strippers contain chemicals that loosen paint from surfaces. These chemicals can harm you if not used properly. Some paint stripping chemicals can irritate the skin and eyes, or cause headaches, drowsiness, nausea, dizziness, or loss of coordination. Some may cause cancer, reproductive problems, or damage of the liver, kidney, or brain. Others catch fire easily. Proper handling and use of paint strippers will reduce your exposure to these chemicals and lessen your health risk.

General Safety Precautions

Paint strippers contain different chemicals, and the potential hazards are different for various products. Each product has specific safety precautions (see the section below on paint stripper types). However, there are some general safety steps to keep in mind when using any paint stripper. If you use paint strippers frequently, it is particularly important that you follow these steps:

1. Always read and follow all the instructions and safety precautions on the label. Do not assume you already know how to use the product. The hazards may be different from one product to another, and the ingredients in individual products often change over time. The label tells you what actions you should take to reduce hazards and the first aid measures to use.
2. Wear chemical-resistant gloves appropriate to the type of stripper being used (see manufacturer's instructions). Common kitchen latex gloves do not provide enough protection.
3. Avoid getting the paint stripper on your skin or in your eyes. Wear protective clothing and goggles appropriate for the project and type of stripper.
4. Use paint strippers outdoors if possible. If you must use them indoors, cross-ventilate by opening all doors and windows. Make sure there is fresh air movement throughout the room. Ventilate the area before, during, and after applying and stripping. Never use any paint stripper in a poorly ventilated area. If work must be done indoors under low ventilation conditions, consider having the work done professionally instead of attempting it yourself.
5. If you work indoors, always work so the stripper fumes are blowing away from you and to the outside. A fan can be used to improve cross-ventilation and to ensure fresh air movement. A fan is particularly important for non-flammable products that evaporate quickly, such as methylene chloride. Electrical sparks from fans may increase the chance of flammable paint strippers fumes to catch fire.
6. Do not use flammable paint strippers near any source of sparks, flame, or high heat. Do not work near gas stoves, kerosene heaters, gas or electric water heaters, gas or electric clothes dryers, gas or electric furnaces, gas or electric space heaters, sanders, buffers, or other electric hand tools. Open flames, cigarettes, matches, lighters, pilot lights, or electric sparks can cause the chemicals in the paint strippers to suddenly catch fire.

7. Only strip paint with chemicals that are marketed as paint strippers. Never use gasoline, lighter fluid, or kerosene to strip paint.
8. Dispose of paint strippers according to the instructions on the label. If you have any questions, ask your local environmental sanitation department about proper disposal.

Types of Paint Strippers

Solvent-based Strippers

Most paint strippers are solvent-based. Solvents dissolve the bond between wood and paint. Solvents also can dissolve other materials, including the latex or rubber of common household or dish washing gloves. Some solvents will irritate or burn the skin. Some solvents may cause serious health effects even if contact does not immediately cause pain. In addition, many solvents evaporate quickly and you can easily inhale them. Inhalation of these solvents can produce health effects immediately or years after exposure.

It is especially important to use paint strippers containing solvents that evaporate quickly either outdoors or in an indoor area with strong fresh air movement. Some paint strippers contain solvents that do not evaporate quickly. When using these strippers indoors, be sure to open windows and doors to provide fresh air movement in and out of the work site. You should always follow the manufacturer's instructions and safety precautions. Use the amount of stripper recommended by the manufacturer to avoid build-up of harmful fumes.

The different types of solvent-based paint strippers and their potential hazards and safety precautions are:

Methylene Chloride (also called dichloromethane, or DCM)

Methylene chloride is the most commonly used chemical in paint strippers. Methylene chloride products come in two varieties. One type is non-flammable, while the other type is flammable. The flammable paint strippers have less methylene chloride but have other flammable chemicals, including acetone, toluene, or methanol.

Methylene chloride causes cancer in laboratory animals. The U.S. Environmental Protection Agency (EPA) and the U.S. Consumer Product Safety Commission (CPSC) consider the chemical to be a potential cause of cancer in humans. Methylene chloride evaporates quickly, and you can inhale it easily. Breathing high levels of methylene chloride over short periods can irritate the eyes, skin, nose, and lungs. It can also cause dizziness, headache, and lack of coordination. Your body changes some inhaled methylene chloride to carbon monoxide. Carbon monoxide lowers the blood's ability to carry oxygen. This can cause problems for people with heart, lung, or blood diseases who use methylene chloride paint strippers indoors without fresh air cross-ventilation. High exposures to methylene chloride for long periods can also cause liver and kidney damage.

It is very important to reduce your exposure to methylene chloride vapors.

It is very important to have a lot of fresh air when using methylene chloride products.

Use methylene chloride paint strippers outdoors if possible. If you must use them indoors, open all doors and windows to ensure that the fresh air is moving in and out of the room.

For indoor use of non-flammable methylene chloride strippers, also use a fan to keep fresh air moving throughout the work area. Electrical sparks from fans may increase the chance of flammable paint strippers fumes to catch fire.

The safest place to use flammable methylene chloride strippers is outdoors away from any source of sparks, flame, or high heat.

Acetone, Toluene and Methanol

These chemicals are commonly used together. All three chemicals evaporate quickly and are very flammable. Breathing high levels of these chemicals can cause a variety of effects, including drowsiness, dizziness, and headache. Breathing high levels of toluene may harm unborn children. Breathing very high levels for a long period may cause brain damage. Toluene and methanol are poisonous if swallowed.

To avoid fire and health problems, it is very important to use products containing these chemicals only in areas with plenty of fresh air.

Do not work near an open flame, pilot lights, or electrical sparks when using flammable paint strippers. Do not use strippers near gas stoves, kerosene heaters, gas or electric water heaters, gas or electric clothes dryers, gas or electric furnaces, gas or electric space heaters, sanders, buffers, or other electric hand tools.

N-methylpyrrolidone (NMP)

Excessive contact with NMP may cause skin swelling, blistering, and burns. These skin reactions may not appear until some time after exposure. N-methylpyrrolidone can readily get into the body through the skin and may cause health problems. NMP may cause reproductive problems and harm to unborn children.

It is very important to wear chemical-resistant gloves and avoid skin contact when using this solvent.

Wash hands immediately after use, even when wearing gloves. Gloves should fit properly and be chemical-resistant. Common kitchen latex gloves do not provide enough protection.

Avoid using this product for extended periods in an enclosed area without open doors or windows to the outside for cross-ventilation.

Dibasic esters (DBE), including dimethyl adipate ester, dimethyl succinate ester, and dimethyl glutarate ester

Much less is known about the possible health effects of these chemicals than about most of the other paint stripping chemicals. Some people using DBE products without fresh air have reported temporary blurred vision. Repeatedly breathing DBE damages the cells lining the nose of laboratory animals. Some strippers include a mixture of DBE products and NMP.

Avoid using this product for extended periods in an enclosed area without open doors or windows to the outside for cross-ventilation.

Use appropriate protective clothing and provide fresh air to the work site when using these products.

Caustoc-based Strippers (Not Flammable)

Caustic Alkalis

Caustic alkalis react with the paint coating and loosen it from the surface. One of the chemicals in this type of stripper is sodium hydroxide (lye). Some people do not use caustic alkalis because caustic products can darken wood and raise the grain. Caustics can cause severe burns to skin and eyes even on short contact. Therefore, be very careful to keep caustic chemicals away from skin and eyes and wear protective clothing. If contact occurs, wash off immediately with cold water. Caustics are also highly toxic if swallowed.

It is very important to avoid skin and eye contact when using caustic alkalis.

Use gloves that fit properly and are appropriate for caustic alkalis.

Wear appropriate protective clothing and goggles when using caustic alkalis.

Other Types of Paint Strippers

Some paint strippers have a citrus smell or make "environmentally friendly" claims. However, these paint strippers may be hazardous despite the smell and environmental claims.

It is important to use appropriate protective clothing and fresh air for cross-ventilation when using these products.

Guidelines by World Health Organisation for Indoor Air Quality: Dampness and Molds

Executive Summary

This document presents World Health Organization (WHO) guidelines for the protection of public health from health risks due to dampness, associated microbial growth and contamination of indoor spaces. The guidelines are based on a comprehensive review and evaluation of the accumulated scientific evidence by a multidisciplinary group of experts studying health effects of indoor air pollutants as well as those specialized in identification of the factors that contribute to microbial growth indoors. Problems of indoor air quality are recognized as important risk factors for human health in both low-income and middle- and high-income countries.

Indoor air is also important because populations spend a substantial fraction of time within buildings. In residences, day-care centres, retirement homes and other special environments, indoor air pollution affects population groups that are particularly vulnerable due to their health status or age. Microbial pollution involves hundreds of species of bacteria and fungi that grow indoors when sufficient moisture is available. Exposure to microbial contaminants is clinically associated with respiratory symptoms, allergies, asthma and immunological reactions.

The microbial indoor air pollutants of relevance to health are widely heterogeneous, ranging from pollen and spores of plants coming mainly from outdoors, to bacteria, fungi, algae and some protozoa emitted outdoors or indoors. They also include a wide variety of microbes and allergens that spread from person to person. There is strong evidence regarding the hazards posed by several biological agents that pollute indoor air; however, the WHO working group convened in October 2006 concluded that the individual species of microbes and other biological agents that are responsible for health effects cannot be identified. This is due to the fact that people are often exposed to multiple agents simultaneously, to complexities in accurately estimating exposure and to the large numbers of symptoms and health outcomes due to exposure. The exceptions include some common allergies, which can be attributed to specific agents, such as house-dust mites and pets.

The presence of many biological agents in the indoor environment is due to dampness and inadequate ventilation. Excess moisture on almost all indoor materials leads to growth of microbes, such as mould, fungi and bacteria, which subsequently emit spores, cells, fragments and volatile organic compounds into indoor air. Moreover, dampness initiates chemical or biological degradation of materials, which also pollutes indoor air. Dampness has therefore been suggested to be a strong, consistent indicator of risk of asthma and respiratory symptoms (e.g. cough and wheeze). The health risks of biological contaminants of indoor air could thus be addressed by considering dampness as the risk indicator.

Health hazards result from a complex chain of events that link penetration of water indoors, excessive moisture to biological growth, physical and chemical degradation, and emission of hazardous biological and chemical agents. The review of scientific evidence that supports these guidelines follows this sequence of events.

The background material for the review was prepared by invited experts and discussed at a WHO working group meeting, convened in Bonn, Germany, 17– 18 October 2007. Sufficient epidemiological evidence is available from studies conducted in different countries and under different climatic conditions to show that the occupants of damp or mouldy buildings, both houses and public buildings, are at increased risk of respiratory symptoms, respiratory infections and exacerbation of asthma. Some evidence suggests increased risks of allergic rhinitis and asthma. Although few intervention studies were available, their results show that remediation of dampness can reduce adverse health outcomes. There is clinical evidence that exposure to mould and other dampness-related microbial agents increases the risks of rare conditions, such as hypersensitivity pneumonitis, allergic alveolitis, chronic rhinosinusitis and allergic fungal sinusitis.

Toxicological evidence obtained in vivo and in vitro supports these findings, showing the occurrence of diverse inflammatory and toxic responses after exposure to micro-organisms isolated from damp buildings, including their spores, metabolites and components. While groups such as atopic and allergic people are particularly susceptible to biological and chemical agents in damp indoor environments, adverse health effects have also been found in nonatopic populations. The increasing prevalences of asthma and allergies in many countries increase the number of people susceptible to the effects of dampness and mould in buildings.

The conditions that contribute to the health risk were summarized as follows. The prevalence of indoor dampness varies widely within and among countries, continents and climate zones. It is estimated to affect 10–50% of indoor environments in Europe, North America, Australia, India and Japan. In certain settings, such as river valleys and coastal areas, the conditions of dampness are substantially more severe than the national averages for such conditions. The amount of water on or in materials is the most important trigger of the growth of micro-organisms, including fungi, actinomycetes and other bacteria. Micro-organisms are ubiquitous. Microbes propagate rapidly wherever water is available. The dust and dirt normally present in most indoor spaces provide sufficient nutrients to support extensive microbial growth. While mould can grow on all materials, selection of appropriate materials can prevent dirt accumulation, moisture penetration and mould growth.

Microbial growth may result in greater numbers of spores, cell fragments, allergens, mycotoxins, endotoxins, β-glucans and volatile organic compounds in indoor air. The causative agents of adverse health effects have not been identified conclusively, but an excess level of any of these agents in the indoor environment is a potential health hazard. Microbial interactions and moisture-related physical and chemical emissions from building materials may also play a role in dampness-related health effects. Building standards and regulations with regard to comfort and health do not sufficiently emphasize requirements for preventing and controlling excess moisture and dampness.

Apart from its entry during occasional events (such as water leaks, heavy rain and flooding), most moisture enters a building in incoming air, including that infiltrating through the building envelope or that resulting from the occupants' activities. Allowing surfaces to become cooler than the surrounding air may result in unwanted condensation. Thermal bridges (such as metal window frames), inadequate insulation and unplanned air pathways, or cold water plumbing and cool parts of air-conditioning units can result in surface temperatures below the dew point of the air and in dampness.

On the basis of this review, the following guidelines were formulated. Persistent dampness and microbial growth on interior surfaces and in building structures should be avoided or minimized, as they may lead to adverse health effects. Indicators of dampness and microbial growth include the presence of condensation on surfaces or in structures, visible mould, perceived mouldy odour and a history of water damage, leakage or penetration. Thorough inspection and, if necessary, appropriate measurements can be used to confirm indoor moisture and microbial growth. As the relations between dampness, microbial exposure and health effects cannot be quantified precisely, no quantitative health-based guideline values or thresholds can be recommended for acceptable levels of contamination with micro-organisms. Instead, it is recommended that dampness and mould-related problems be prevented. When they occur, they should be remediated because they increase the risk of hazardous exposure to microbes and chemicals.

Well-designed, well-constructed, well-maintained building envelopes are critical to the prevention and control of excess moisture and microbial growth, as they prevent thermal bridges and the entry of liquid or vapour-phase water. Management of moisture requires proper control of temperatures and ventilation to avoid excess humidity, condensation on surfaces and excess moisture in materials. Ventilation should be distributed effectively throughout spaces, and stagnant air zones should be avoided. Building owners are responsible for providing a healthy workplace or living environment free of excess moisture and mould, by ensuring proper building construction and maintenance.

The occupants are responsible for managing the use of water, heating, ventilation and appliances in a manner that does not lead to dampness and mould growth. Local recommendations for different climatic regions should be updated to control dampness-mediated microbial growth in buildings and to ensure desirable indoor air quality. Dampness and mould may be particularly prevalent in poorly maintained housing for low-income people. Remediation of the conditions that lead to adverse exposure should be given priority to prevent an additional contribution to poor health in populations who are already living with an increased burden of disease.

The guidelines are intended for worldwide use, to protect public health under various environmental, social and economic conditions, and to support the achievement of optimal indoor air quality. They focus on building characteristics that prevent the occurrence of adverse health effects associated with dampness or mould. The guidelines pertain to various levels of economic development and different climates, cover all relevant population groups and propose feasible approaches for reducing health risks due to dampness and microbial contamination. Both private and public buildings (e.g. offices and nursing homes) are covered, as dampness and mould are risks everywhere.

Settings in which there are particular production processes and hospitals with high-risk patients or sources of exposure to pathogens are not, however, considered. While the guidelines provide objectives for indoor air quality management, they do not give instructions for achieving those objectives. The necessary action and indicators depend on local technical conditions, the level of development, human capacities and resources. The guidelines recommended by WHO acknowledge this heterogeneity. In formulating policy targets, governments should consider their local circumstances and select actions that will ensure achievement of their health objectives most effectively.

Guidelines by National Safety Council

Sick Building Syndrome

What is Sick Building Syndrome?

Sick Building Syndrome (SBS) is a situation in which occupants of a building experience acute health effects that seem to be linked to time spent in a building, but no specific illness or cause can be identified. The complaints may be localized in a particular room or zone, or may be widespread throughout the building.

Frequently, problems result when a building is operated or maintained in a manner that is inconsistent with its original design or prescribed operating procedures. Sometimes indoor air problems are a result of poor building design or occupant activities.

What are the Symptoms of SBS?

Building occupants complain of symptoms associated with acute discomfort. These symptoms include headaches; eye, nose, and throat irritation; a dry cough; dry or itchy skin; dizziness and nausea; difficulty in concentrating; fatigue; and sensitivity to odors. With SBS, no clinically defined disease or specific chemical or biological contaminant can be determined as the cause of the symptoms. Most of the complainants feel relief soon after leaving the building.

SBS reduces worker productivity and may also increase absenteeism.

What causes SBS?

While specific causes of SBS remain unknown, the following have been cited as contributing factors to Sick Building Syndrome. These elements may act in combination or may supplement other complaints such as inadequate temperature, humidity, or lighting.

- Chemical contaminants from outdoor sources: Outdoor air that enters a building can also be a source of indoor pollution. Pollutants from motor vehicle exhausts, plumbing vents, and building exhausts (bathrooms and kitchens) can enter the building through poorly located air intake vents, windows, and other openings. Combustion by-products can also enter a building from a nearby garage.
- Chemical contaminants from indoor sources: Most indoor air pollution comes from sources inside the building. For example, adhesives, upholstery, carpeting, copy machines, manufactured wood products, cleaning agents and pesticides may emit volatile organic compounds (VOCs) including formaldehyde. Research shows that some VOCs can cause chronic and acute health effects at high concentrations, and some are known carcinogens. Low to moderate levels of multiple VOCs may also produce acute reactions in some individuals. Environmental tobacco smoke and combustion products from stoves, fireplaces, and unvented space heaters all can put chemical contaminants into the air.

Information and recommendations are compiled from sources believed to be reliable. The National Safety Council makes no guarantee as to and assumes no responsibility for the correctness, sufficiency or completeness of such information or recommendations. Other or additional safety measures may be required under particular circumstances.

- **Biological contaminants**: Biological contaminants include pollen, bacteria, viruses, and molds. These contaminants can breed in stagnant water that has accumulated in humidifiers, drain pans, and ducts, or where water has collected on ceiling tiles, insulation, or carpet. Biological contaminants can cause fever, chills, cough, chest tightness, muscle aches, and allergic reactions. One indoor air bacterium, Legionella, has caused both Pontiac Fever and Legionnaire's Disease.
- Inadequate ventilation: In the 1970s the oil embargo led building designers to make buildings more airtight, with less outdoor air ventilation, in order to improve energy efficiency. These reduced ventilation rates have been found to be, in many cases, inadequate to maintain the health and comfort of building occupants.

What are the Solutions to Sick Building Syndrome?

Solutions to SBS problems usually include combinations of the following measures:

- Increasing the ventilation rates and air distribution is often a cost-effective means of reducing indoor pollutant levels. At a minimum, heating, ventilating, and air conditioning (HVAC) systems should be designed to meet ventilation standards in local building codes. Make sure that the system is operated and maintained to ensure that the design ventilation rates are attained. If possible, the HVAC system should be operated to the American Society of Heating, Refrigerating and Air-Conditioning Engineers (ASHRAE) Standard 62-1989. If there are strong pollutant sources, air may need to be vented directly to the outside. This method is especially recommended to remove pollutants that accumulate in specific areas such as restrooms, copy rooms, and printing facilities.
- Removal or modification of the pollutant source is the most effective approach to solving a known source of an indoor air quality problem when this solution is practicable. Ways to do this include routine maintenance of HVAC systems; replacing water-stained ceiling tiles and carpets; banning smoking or providing a separately ventilated room; venting contaminant source emissions to the outdoors; using and storing paints, solvents, pesticides, and adhesives in closed containers in well-ventilated areas; using those pollutant sources in periods of low or no occupancy; and allowing time for building materials in new or remodeled areas to off-gas pollutants before occupancy.
- Air cleaning has some limitations, but it can be a useful addition to source control and ventilation. Air filters are only effective at removing some, not all, of the pollution.

- Education and communication are important parts of any air quality management program. When everyone associated with the building, from occupants to maintenance, fully understands the issues and communicates with each other they can work more effectively together to prevent and solve problems.

Guidelines by Indian Green Building Council

6 Steps to Prevent Indoor Air Pollution in Your Home

Studies show that many times indoor pollution takes more of a toll on your health than outdoor pollution. As we walk through our homes, the air turbulence created by our moving bodies stirs up a combination of dust and debris that can be very irritating to the lungs.

Indoor Air Pollution and Irritants

Human skin particles, pollen, and smoke are all part of this bothersome brew of irritants. The most irritating are dust mites. Dust mites are microscopic creatures that feed on dust especially flakes of skin. Household cleaners and pesticides are full of chemicals. People are even bothered by low levels of these compounds. Ironically, indoor air is now recognized as being full of many of the same chemicals we've spent so much time reducing outdoors. Another common source of indoor air pollution is dry-cleaned clothes, which emit a number of chemicals that may be harmful. Fortunately, homeowners these days have a wide range of options that can help them breathe more easily and comfortably in the home.

1. Reduce and alter indoor chemical use Pay close attention to the labels on household products. If possible switch to natural products that contain fewer toxic chemicals. When you do need to use a stronger chemical, use it sparingly and follow all the precautions explained on the label.
2. Air out dry-cleaned items Don't immediately store dry-cleaned items in a closet. Take the plastic off and allow your clothing to air out for a day or two in a space with good air circulation. Then, recover the items with plastic and store them in a closet.
3. Use more sophisticated furnace filters The traditional furnace air filter isn't designed to clean air. Its only function is to keep large particles, like hair and debris, from damaging the furnace blower. These larger particles are rarely the source of human breathing difficulty. Now there are new, more elaborate filters on the market that trap enough particulate matter to help humans breathe better. In general, the more costly the filter, the more dust it snags out of the airflow. Costing anywhere from $7 to $100, sophisticated filters can pull out up to five times as much dust as traditional filters.

4. Install an electronic air cleaner Electronic air cleaners can extract 30 times as much dust as ordinary filters, but they cost a lot more. In fact, a professionally installed air cleaner costs $500 to $700. While this is a substantial amount of money, it's worth every penny if it offers significant breathing relief to one or more people in your household. If the price is too steep for you, portable units can be purchased for far less. Of course, the smaller units clean just the air in one room-much like a window air conditioner cools only one room. Electronic air cleaners only need to be cleaned once a year or so because they incinerate the trapped dust.
5. Open the windows Don't keep your home tightly sealed all of the time. Years ago homes weren't nearly as insulated as they are today. However, one drawback to this is that indoor toxins also get sealed inside. It's important to air out your home regularly by opening windows and using fans to draw outside fresh air inside. Installing an attic or whole house fan is a great way to bring a big breath of fresh air indoors.

6. Add plants to your home Plants can do a great job of helping to remove the indoor toxins from home. And, some plants work harder at it than others. A few that have been shown to work well: Boston fern, spider plant, English ivy, areca palm, and peace lillies. A good rule of thumb is two plants per hundred square feet.

Guidelines by Griha-Adarsh

Building and Site Design Elements

Site Inventory Characteristic #1
Geographical Latitude and Micro-Climatic factors such as Wind Loads

1. Building Layout for Solar Orientation

The ideal case would be to have a compact, square plan with perfect alignment with the cardinal directions. However, in less than ideal cases, the optimum orientation for buildings in the tropics is with their longer axes along east-west At a site level, the orientation of the building is determined by adjacent buildings and landforms. High-rise buildings in close proximity of a proposed building can compromise the daylight access of the interior spaces, prevent natural ventilation, and re-radiate absorbed heat towards the proposed building, leading to increased energy consumption. This can be prevented easily through proper, site-responsive orientation of the building. In Part 8, Table 3 of the National Building Code, the values of the total solar radiation (direct plus diffused) incident on various surfaces of buildings in $W/m^2/day$ for summer and winter seasons is provided. It is judicious to avoid the orientations with highest solar radiation incident and plan the building layout accordingly.

Location of Green and Pave Areas

Green areas such as trees and shrubs should be planted in response to climatic and site requirements. Trees can serve as filters to cool prevailing hot winds. They can also be used to shelter a building from harsh cold/hot winds. Paved areas should be kept away from the building to prevent heat island impacts. They should be minimized to retain the site permeability. Conversely, gravel could be used as against tar/asphalt to retain the permeability of the site.

2. Location of Windows

Windows should be located along tie southern and northern facades with adequate provision for shading to prevent heat gain. Well shaded windows on the southern facade can enable passive heating in winter and shaded daylight spaces in summer.

Biodiversity

An existing green area shall have several species of flora and fauna living in a delicate balance with nature. This contributes to several aspects such as automatic disease control through natural food chains, as well as checking pests. This should be retained and an attempt should be made to enhance this aspect of the site.

3. Entrances and Loading Docks

Building entrances should be positioned away from the direct impacts of the local site and climatic conditions. Sheltering them from winds and direct radiation can ensure that the building and its occupants are provided with an adequately sheltered zone to enter the building through.

Selection of Vegetation and Integration with the Native Landscape

Vegetation is the key element that supports the biodiversity of an area/ site. Exotic/imported species actually contribute to the mass extinction of several native species of flora and fauna. Vegetation species should be native to the agro-climatic zone where the building is proposed. Also note aspects of deciduous/ evergreen nature of trees tor seasonal solar control. Deciduous trees can prevent direct solar radiation from impacting the building in summer, while allowing radiation through in winter due to leaf shedding.

4. Location of Air Inlets

There are global winds and localized winds. Both should be studied before providing air inlets for ventilation purposes. Spacing of buildings and their mutual distances must also be optimized to induce natural ventilation in all the buildings of a region. High-density, high-rise buildings disrupt winds by creating wind shadow areas to distances up to 15 times their height. They also halve the wind velocity. So adequate spacing between buildings must be provided to ensure equal access to natural ventilation in all buildings. An air quality study must also be conducted to see whether the air is suitable for ventilation purposes.

Use of Landscape Elements as Buffer Zones

Trees can act as buffers for hot winds, noise, pollution, and so on, and the landscape strategy should account for this. Single or double rows of trees at distances of 0.7 to 1.5 metres should be used to create shelter belts, and a mixture of species is recommended." The distance between adjacent, parallel rows should be at least two metres for effectiveness. Also, elements such as hillocks can be used (if existing) or created (if there is excavated soil from the site) as obstacles for noise. Water bodies can also be used for evaporative cooling if located in the requisite part of the site for maximum benefit.

5. Architectural Elevations

Elevations must respond to the local climatic conditions. Elements such as balconies, verandahs, and external corridors can serve effectively as external shading devices and prevent heat gain in the summers. The elevation can be broken up into smaller elements such that the overall surface area exposed to direct solar radiation is reduced. Local traditional architectural practices often relied extensively on such interventions, therefore local/regional trends should be studied and understood to help respond better to the regional climate.

Site Inventory Characteristic #2– Topography and Adjacent Landforms

1. Building Proportions

The surface to volume ratio and the perimeter to area ratio largely determine its potential to exploit solar passive design features effectively. Both these ratios, if kept to a minimum in hot climates lead to an efficient design. In cold climates, high surface to volume (s/v) ratio can be coupled with attached sun spaces, or solaria, to capture heat and passively heat the interior spaces. Thus, a compact plan with properly zoned interior spaces (with buffer spaces such as stairwells and toilets on the sides of maximum heat gain) can generate a very efficient and low-energy architecture.

Gravity-fed Sewer Lines

Sewer lines can be so designed as complement the natural slope of the land and contours. This can ensure that no pumping energy shall be required to carry sewage across the site and into the municipal sewers.

2. Wind Loads

Keeping in view global and local wind patterns, the opening in a building can be designed to curtail or exploit the winds on site. Often due to adjacent wind forms, pockets of very high wind pressure are created or vice versa. Windows and their shades (such as vertical louvers) or other building elements such as walls and trees can be used to deflect winds towards or away from a building as required.

Landfilling

Altering the levels of the site via cutting and filling activities must be done to the minimum and very judiciously. This is because altering the slope often leads to increased flow of water and erosion of soil. This requires further construction of appropriate drainage interventions to contain and control the storm/sewage water. This may also compromise the bearing capacity of the soil over a period of time and lead to land-slides and slippages.

3. Architectural Elevations

Topography and adjacent built/natural forms can often require elevations to be treated very differently in comparison to what the climate demands. If an adjacent building is blocking the proposed building's right to light or ventilation, larger windows/air-inlets may need to be provided on a facade that ordinarily would not permit the same due to energy considerations. Thus, the localized architectural elevations and facade details should also respond to the micro-climatic/site conditions.

Natural site features for Rain/Storm Water Drainage

Sustainable urban drainage strategy (SUDS) requires maximum utilization of the natural site features to integrate as benign a sewage management system as possible on site. This requires retaining as many natural features as possible and trying to design an architectural intervention that does the least to compromise/ drastically alter the existing conditions on site. The architectural design can be made to respond to the existing site conditions to the maximum possible extent. Please note that this also requires minimum economic investment and minimum expenditure on energy consumption over the life cycle of the building.

4. Drainage Strategies

Drainage strategies should be based on sustainable urban drainage systems or SUDS. Conventional systems direct all the water during heavy downpour into a drainage system, often leading to flooding or clogging. SUDS ensures that the flow is attenuated using natural means so as to slow the flow as also employ natural systems that can purify and filter the water. This water can then be suitably used on the site to cater to the building's demand. These often cost lesser money to construct and are can be designed in a manner as to not require connection to a main city sewer system. (Eg. Swales, Soakaways, Holding ponds, pervious surfaces, optimally-designed pervious pavement systems, etc.)

Location of Groundwater Detention Ponds

Detention ponds can affect the flow of surface water and its run-off from the site in consideration, by catching and holding the water and slowly releasing it into either a SUDS or a conventional sewage system. The location of the ponds should complement the natural slope and should be so located as to effectively hold water from the entire site over the period of discharge into the drainage systems/SUDS. The lowest points of the site should be selected for the location of the detention ponds, and the number of ponds should be decided via detailed calculations based on the run-off coefficients of the site and the surfaces on site.

Site Inventory Characteristic #3– Solar Access

1. Building Position for Daylighting

In order to reduce dependency on energy intensive systems for lighting and ventilation, buildings must be planned in a manner as to allow maximum ingress of natural light and permit natural ventilation as far as possible in all occupied spaces. Daylighting can be maximized with an optimal visible sky component (SC) in all occupied spaces. This is possible only if the windows opening into the occupied spaces are free of any obstructions that may block a clear view of the sky from them. This also includes adjacent buildings, trees, and other elements. Under ideal conditions, the lowest floor windows should subtend an angle not greater than 22.5 degrees with the top of an adjacent building/object. This angle also ensures an ideal distance for sound natural ventilation.

Location of energy-efficient features such as Solar Pond

Features such as solar ponds can help store the radiant energy of the sun as heat, in a manner as to be able to use it for various applications such hot-water generation and electricity generation. Such features are also most effective if they are located at a part of the site where they encounter minimum obstruction from other buildings and natural elements on the site. The clearer their view of the sky, the more they are likely to receive as direct solar radiation and the more shall be the stored heat in them. Thus, such features must be located on the site in a careful manner so as to ensure no shadows or obstructions during installation as well as over their entire life cycle.

2. Photovoltaics

For positioning solar photovoltaic panels for generation of energy on-site, it is imperative that a shadow-free area be identified with an orientation appropriate for optimal generation and efficiency of the solar panel. It is determined as a rule of thumb that the ideal orientation for optimal performance of a solar cell is at an angle equivalent to the latitude of the place where it is being installed.

Placement of selective species of trees (such as deciduous trees on the south of the site)

As is clear from the National Building Code 2005 (Part 8 building services, Section 01 - Lighting and Ventilation, Table 3 - Direct and diffused solar radiation values for various orientations) some parts of a building facade need to be protected from the harsh glare of direct sunlight and other parts need to be shaded only seasonally. Among the most economical ways of doing this is by an appropriate planting/landscape design strategy that identifies specific trees for specific orientations. Deciduous trees planted on the south side can ensure that the building spaces are shaded through the harsh summers, but get adequate sunlight for passive heating during winters when they shed their leaves. Similarly, having evergreen trees on the east and west facade can ensure glare-free natural lighting in the spaces in a particular orientation of the building.

3. Solar Passive Techniques

Architectural design interventions can significantly impact a building's energy requirement. Features such as Window to wall ratio (the ratio of the total glazed/ window area to the entire wall area in that specific orientation), solar chimneys, attached sun spaces, trompe walls, and so on, are extremely site-specific and must be located on orientations of the building that complement the local site conditions. Passive heating features should be located such that they absorb maximum solar radiation though the day.

4. Construction of Walls

The height and distance of walls from a building can impact and influence the ability of the building to exploit natural light and ventilation. Often it is observed that site boundary walls are built up to 3 metres or 4.5 metres. As mentioned earlier, impermeable obstructions such as solid walls can create wind-shadow areas up to a distance equivalent to 8-10 times the height of the wall. This can seriously compromise the uniformity of wind pressure and natural ventilation on the building site. When the winds converge back on to the ground they tend to create eddies that can further give rise to pockets of high/low wind pressure. This further impacts the comfort of the people on the site. So walls must be built taking into account the likelihood of its impact on the site and its surrounding areas.

5. Selection of Building Materials and Finishing

Building materials and finishes can help enhance the performance of the building with respect to solar passive features, or vice-versa. All building materials (as with all elements in nature) have the inherent capacity to absorb, reflect or transmit heat to varying degrees. This impacts the thermal comfort of the occupants of the building and resultantly the energy demand of the building. The external materials selected for a building must be done carefully so as to ensure minimum transmission of heat through the facade, while simultaneously reducing the heat reflected to the surrounding structures and natural features. The light reflected of neighbouring buildings can also impact the visual comfort requirements of one's building by increasing glare conditions. This must be avoided.

Site Inventory Characteristic #4– Air Movement Patterns

1. Placement of Wind Towers

Passive cooling/ventilation elements should be located in the directions that exploit maximum wind ingress. Wind towers need to capture the hot summer winds so must be oriented in a complementary direction. They should also be located in a manner as to not be impacted by neighbouring/ structures. In other words, they should not be in the wind-shadow areas of neighbouring developments or trees.

Site layout of Building Structures to Trap Wind for Ventilation

The wind flow through a site is influenced by the following features:

- Immediate topography
- Vegetation (trees, shrubs, and so on) on the topography
- Adjacent landforms around the site
- Adjacent built forms around the site
- The building layout on the site itself

Thus, building footprints must be planned out in a manner as to enhance the prevalent site conditions and the micro-climate. Buildings can help channel wind-flow in a particular direction as may be required on site. They can also funnel the wind and increase/decrease its pressure. So buildings must be planned in a manner that not only enhances the conditions on site, but also ensures that the surrounding developments get their share of natural winds on their developments as well.

2. Location of Fenestration on the basis of Pressure Differentials

Operable/open-able windows that are designed for natural ventilation should be so positioned as to balance the pressure differential that may exist on the site due to surrounding conditions. In case the windows are not perpendicular to the prevailing wind direction, the windows and window features such as louvres (vertical or horizontal) can be used to channel winds into an internal space by deflection. Similarly, they can also be designed to shelter the window from high-velocity winds. Thus, they must be designed appropriately.

3. Passive Solar Cooling Design

Passive solar cooling features include shading devices, plantation plans, solar chimneys, earth air tunnels (earth air heat exchangers). The buildings must be planned and laid out to incorporate as many of such features as is possible on the site and ensure that the comfort requirements of the building are met through minimum reliance on energy intensive technologies such as refrigerant-based HVAC systems.

Site Inventory Characteristic #5–
Parcel Shape and Access with Adjacent Land use and Buildings

1. Planning for the Capacity to Accommodate the Proposed Development

Density of development should ideally be determined by the capacity required to accommodate an accurately estimated number of people, with a small provision for future expansion. It is common to construct large buildings on speculation and then sell them for purely commercial benefit This can lead to oversized systems, excess use of materials, and larger environmental impact and depletion than is actually required. Such an approach must be avoided to ensure healthy living conditions and energy security for future generations.

Marking the Potential Access Points that Do Not Burden the Lower Density or Adjacent Land use

The National Building Code, Part 3, under the Development Control Rules and General Building Requirements, slates, 'In no case, development on plots shall be permitted unless it is accessible by a public street of width no less than 6 metres.' Larger building developments require a minimum road width of 12 metres. It also states that In no case shall the means of access be lesser in width than the internal access ways in layouts and subdivisions'. This should be followed.

Site Inventory Characteristic #6– Neighbouring or Proposed Future Developments

1. Design Flexibility for Future Extension

Future extensions may be carried out on one's own site or on neighbouring site. Provisions should be left for both expansion types. This implies that just as we would not want to build on a site where the neighbouring developments compromise our rights to natural light and ventilation, so should we take the responsibility of ensuring adequate inter-building spacing and overall site planning as to ensure adequate light and air for the future buildings to come.

Location of Utility and Infrastructure for Future Extension

Similar to design flexibility for the future, we must also ensure adequate provisions to ensure easy extension of utilities and infrastructure on our site. This should take into account aspects such as increase in occupancy, increase in built-up area, climate change related impacts (increased rainfall, or drought), and so on.

About the Authors

Prof. Dr. Bharat Bhushan Puri

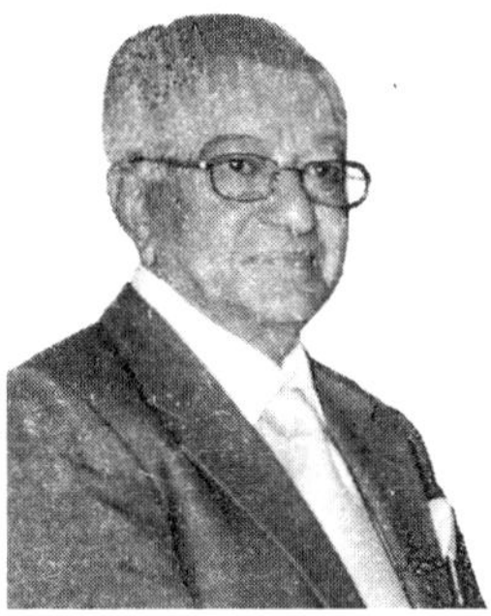

Sr. Architect, Author, Research Scholar and Senior Vastu Advisor

Prof. Dr. B.B. Puri is a multifaceted personality and he is a Senior Practicing Architect, Research Scholar, Author and Vastu Advisor. He is associated with numerous professional organizations. His achievements highlight his versatile character.

Prof. Puri has added a new research dimension and scientific approach to Vedic Culture making it a modern concept in the Vedic Philosophy.

Prof. Puri's creative ability in the field of Architecture has earned him many commendations from Dr. Zakir Hussain, Shri V.V. Giri, Dr. Giani Zail Singh, Dr. Shankar Dayal Sharma, and Shri. K. R. Narayanan, Former Presidents of India. He was also honoured with a shield and testimonial by Smt. Indira Gandhi, and Shri. Rajiv Gandhi, Former Prime Ministers of India.

He has travelled widely and has participated in and headed many National and International Conferences and Seminars. He is the recipient of numerous awards and notes of appreciation from renowned personalities. He has been honoured with the **Bharat Gaurav Award** (1996), **Bhaskar Award** (1997). A biographical note on Prof. Puri was featured in **India's Who's Who** (1978) and **Prominent Personalities of India** (1979). He has been conferred with **The Gem of India Award** (1998), **Business Initiative Development Award** (1998), **National Excellency Award** (1999), **Health Excellence Award** (2000), **The International Academician Fellowship Award** (2002), **Master of Wisdom-National Award** (2008) by Media Trust of India, **Vedic Signature Award** (2008).

On 27th May, 2009, the M.G.I and R.T.I., Moka–Mauritius awarded **The Light of East Award**. He was also the recipient of **Distinguished Service Award** (2010) by Geriatric Society of India, **Life Time Achievement Award** by World Management Congress (2011), **Social Responsibility Award** by Bharat Nirman (2013). He also received an Award from International Congress on Geriatric Care on 16th November, 2013; another **Award of Honour for** National Seminar on Vaastu Science (2014).

He has been honoured with **The Millennium Award** and a Gold Medal at the Millennium World Congress (2000) for his lifetime achievements.

Prof. Puri has written more than 120 books. The then Hon'ble President of India had released his popular books titled **'Vedic Architecture and Art of Living'** and **'Applied Vastu Shastra in Modern Architecture'** at Rashtrapati Bhawan. His latest books titled **'Vastu Science for 21st Century to Enjoy the Gift of Nature'**, **'The Ageless Mind'**, **'Mass Scale Housing for Hot Climate'**, **'The Art of Blissful Living, Spiritual Laws of Vedic Philosophy'**, **'Life Before Death'** and **'In Search of God–One Soul Many Gods'** have been well received.

Prof. Puri is the Founder and Chairman of–

- **Grover & Puri** (Architects since, 1960)
- **Research Institute of Vedic Culture** (N.G.O)
- **Vastu Research Centre**
- **Indian Institute of Building Technology** (IIBT)
- **Design Gurukul** (An Institution for Professionals)
- **Vastu Kala Academy** (College of Architecture)
- **The Institution of Vastu Science** (India)
- Trustee, Word Academy of Spiritual Sciences
- H.O.D. Occult Science, Zoroastrian College, Mumbai
- Vice President, Geriatric Society of India
- **Society of Love & Live in Peace** (So Lip)

Visiting Professor–

- CPWD Training Institute, Govt. of India
- ALTC, Govt. of India

- Zoroastrian College, Mumbai
- M.G.I. Moka, Mauritius
- Tribhuvan University, Kathmandu, Nepal

Prof. Puri is the Life Member of–

- Council of Architecture
- International Council of Consultants
- Indian Building Congress
- India International Centre
- Indian Council of Social Welfare
- Institute of Chartered Engineers
- A.M.I.C.E. India and U.S.A.
- India Habitat Centre
- Engineering Council of India
- Construction Industry Development Council
- Construction Industry Arbitration Council
- Temple of Understanding

His contact details:

W–151, G.K. Part I, New Delhi-110048
Ph.: 011-29242224 Mob.: 9999966351
E-mail: dr.bbpuri@yahoo.com
Website: www.profpurivrc.com

Dr. R.M. Mehra

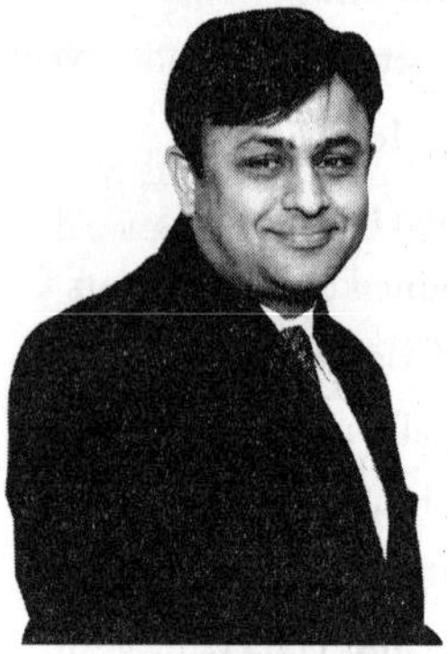

Ph.D and D.Sc

Dr. R.M. Mehra is an Interior Designer, Scientific Vastu Expert, Sick Building Expert, Colour Consultant, Research Scholar and an Author. He is among the very few Research Scholars, Ph.D and D.Sc in the field of Interior Design and Scientific Vastu. He is the Director of Building Doctors and Design Gurukul. He is the Research Director of RIVC (NGO Trust). He is a member of the Institute of Indian Interior Designers. He is both an Educationalist and a Consultant. He has trained lots of Interior Designers, Architects and Vastu consultants. He is one of the few experts who pursues Sick Building Syndrome and Scientific Vastu with instruments. Some of his prominent clients include **Birla Group of Companies, Reliance Group of Companies, Real Tech Builders, Uppals Group, Low Price Publications, Excel Books, JIMS, Design Forum of Architects, Sumitomitsui Constructions, Lakhani Group of Companies** etc. Building Doctors, a member of Indian Green Building Council, provides Sick Building and Premium Scientific Vastu consultation services.

Dr. Mehra has done his post-doctoral research in Vasteriology and Interior Psychology. He is among the very few consultants who practices and teaches the amazing secret world of colours and has used multi-functional aspects of colours in interiors, healing, meditation and vastu science and is doing extensive research on chromatics. He has introduced Colours as a professional specialization for various courses. Design Gurukul conducts various specialization programs in the area of Building Sciences. Dr. Mehra has introduced a new specialization field, **Vasteriology** (Science of Vastu, Interiors and Psychology). It is a micro branch of Vastu, concentrating on elementary aspects of Vastu and Interiors through the perspective of human psychology.

Dr. Mehra has presented various technical papers and has received numerous awards of appreciation. He has been honoured with a **Gold Medal** and citation at the Millennium World Congress in 2005. He has been given the **Special Award of Honour** and **Speakers Special Award** by the Zoroastrian College, Mumbai in 2006. He has also been awarded **"First Healthy Home Consultant Award"** by the XXth National Medicos Congress, Hoshiarpur, Punjab. He has been honoured with an **Award of Excellence in Research and Professional Services** by the Minister of Culture and Tourism, Smt. Ambika Soni in 2009. Recently, he was bestowed by **Award of Excellence for Research and Outstanding Services as a Guide** by RIVC, **Certificate of Excellence** from Rotary Club, Ghaziabad, **Speakers Special Award** and **Silver Jublilee Award** from Zoroastrian College, Mumbai.

His book **'The Healthy Office'** is based on creating healthy environment in an office. Mr. Mantytsky, Russian Counsel in Mumbai released the book in 2006. His recent book **'I Thought My Home Was Healthy?'** is based on creating healthy and vastu-friendly interiors in a home. Smt. Sheila Dikshit, the then Chief Minister of Delhi, released the book in 2009. Both the books have been well received.

His contact details:

N–104, 2B, 2nd Floor,
Kirti Nagar, New Delhi
Ph.: 011-64582627 Mob.: 9911184404
Email: dr.rmmehra@rediffmail.com
Website: www.buildingdoctors.in/www.colourexperts.org